THE OTHER SIDE OF THE GURNEY

Stories and Reflections of a 911 Paramedic

Connie Carson-Romano

ISBN: 1508451184
ISBN 13: 9781508451181

*This book is dedicated to my husband, Michael, for his love and belief in me.
It is also dedicated to my three children,
Tom, Chris, and Crystal,
who lived through these times with me and gave me the courage to continue.*

CONTENTS

INTRODUCTION

This book began as a book about my life as an EMT and paramedic. For me it was cathartic to put into words the drama, trauma, laughter, and sadness evoked by those years in the field. I have moved on since I began writing down these stories, expanded my education, and changed the focus of my practice. The stories follow my evolution and include a few experiences I had working as a registered nurse.

The majority of the stories in this book are of my own experiences in the field of medicine. Some are sad. Some are funny. Some are feel-good stories. They are all true to the best of my recollection. When coworkers and friends found out I was writing these stories down, I was inundated with stories of their own telling. My only requirement was that the stories were true. Some of the stories did not make the cut, but of the ones that did, I hope the retelling is to the satisfaction of those who shared them.

Some of the names and locations of the people in this book have been changed. That is for not only their protection but mine as well since not all of the stories presented are politically correct. The HIPAA privacy laws were not yet on the books when most of these stories happened, but I have rewritten the placement and nonpertinent facts of some of these stories to cover any violation of legalities.

Some of the stories may offend you. I don't apologize for that. These are true stories. I can only say that if you are too offended, don't read the book.

I have changed the title of this book many times during its evolution. The original title was *The Accidental Heroes* and was written for all of the people I have known that spent their lives working in medicine. Not many got into medicine wanting to be a hero. Most of us just liked people. We were given the gift of reacting to stressful situations calmly and the intelligence to learn the skills necessary to help resolve some of the problems presented. Because of that, we were invited into the homes and lives of people during the most stressful and frightening times imaginable. That is an honor of the highest sort. Thank-yous are rare and definitely not expected but so welcome when they do come. We are heroic only by the hand of fate and our choice of occupation. It is very humbling to witness the most intimate events in the lives of people. There are times that it wrenches the heart to see the hurt, anguish, and fear of the people who seek us out. Sometimes we get to share in their joy when things go right. And occasionally the humor of the situations is...well, just uncontrollably funny.

Another one of the other titles that had its moment during the development of this manuscript was *The Worst Thing Ever.* That one was borne because when you work in emergency medicine, one of the first questions people ask is, what is the worst call/thing/injury you ever saw? That one didn't last long as I realized that the worst thing I ever saw had to do with the state of mind I was in at the time and the emotions that I held latent inside. Therefore, the worst thing I ever saw had more to do with my emotional response to the situation than the gore or graphic descriptions could convey. I did, however, identify some of the situations I wrote about as having been episodes that affected me deeply. And, after twenty years of twenty-four-hour shifts with eight to twenty calls per shift, these are the stories that have registered in my memory.

Another aspect that has changed since the inception of these stories is my ability to see the other side. We all get older, and the lifelong throws of the dice deliver us eventually into a spot where we too seek help from others. So I have included in these stories peeks into my own life from the other side of the gurney.

I initially just wrote down the stories as I experienced them but have since inserted short examinations of feelings and lessons I learned along the way. I don't think I realized the value of my emotional response to these stories until I was old enough to appreciate my own wisdom. That is one of the real values of getting older.

Stories about medicine, especially emergency medicine, will always be popular for the same reason that we all (whether we admit it or not) look at accidents on the side of the road. We all fear the worst that can happen and wish it doesn't happen to us. I hope that in addition to satisfying that desire to know, my stories will also help you understand that there are people out there who will help when it does happen. Because eventually we will all face an episode just like those in this book.

BEGINNINGS

The sun was warm on my arm as I drove my beat-up old blue van down the dirt road to the corner store. A hazy phloem of dust crowded my rearview mirror as I reflected. Sunday morning was my time. I would put the coffee on to brew and then drive down to the little store on the corner for a newspaper. After buying a newspaper, I would visit with Gina, the clerk, catching up on all the local gossip before driving home with my coffee and paper to my porch swing, which looked out over the high plains of New Mexico. The sun and my cup of steaming coffee would warm me and revitalize me for another week; then the kids would wake up, and my day would get started. Reading the Sunday paper with that cup of coffee was mandatory for the week that would ensue.

That day didn't seem any different from any other day, but the focus of my life was about to change dramatically.

I purchased my paper and tucked it under my arm, enjoying a leisurely chat with Gina about who was doing what with whom and the general moral decline of the people in our little town when the glass door was thrown open, and a middle-aged woman flew into the store. Her eyes were dilated with terror, and her cheeks glowed bright red. "Help," she begged, gasping for breath. "There's been an accident."

I tossed my treasured Sunday paper on the counter and told Gina to call for help. "I'll go see if I can do anything," I said, following the frantic woman out the door.

The little store fronted a two-lane state highway, and as I exited, my eyes focused on a full-size pickup with a crumpled front end that was sitting at an awkward angle on the highway. Two elderly people and a third man wearing a plaid cowboy shirt stood on the side of the road looking down into the field. I started toward them when the woman from the store grabbed my arm. "No," she said. "There!" My gaze followed her pointing finger about fifty feet down the road and off the embankment to a section of displaced barbed-wire fence that protected the cattle from the highway and vice-versa. Tangled in the fence like a crushed fly in a spider's web was a small car. I knew it had taken quite an impact to send the little car so far from the road. "He's not moving," the woman holding my arm whispered. Neither was anyone else.

Wishing I had worn something more than the flimsy sandals that covered my feet, I plowed through the tumbleweed toward the mangled car. The car was crushed badly on the driver's side, and at first I didn't see anyone in it. My hands were gripping the windowsill before I saw the elderly man in the car lying sideways across the front seats, where he had been thrown by the impact.

"Mister, are you O.K.?" Even as the words left my mouth, I knew that he wasn't. His eyes were half-open, and his breath eased out of his mouth and down onto the front seat of the little car in a bubbly pink froth.

I tugged at the car door, but it wouldn't budge. Running to the passenger side, I squeezed myself into the window to reach for a pulse. Again, the useless words passed my lips. "Mister, are you O.K.?" My heart sank as I frantically reached for the other side of his neck and hopefully a pulse. I prayed that maybe I had just missed it. But the absence of a pulse and the slow escape of air told me I had to do something fast. Pulling myself from the window, I turned to look for help. A crowd of people had gathered on the road by the truck, but no one was moving in my direction. "I need help down here now," I yelled. The man wearing the plaid shirt started in my direction. Turning back to the car and bracing my foot on the rear door, I managed to wrench the driver's door loose from its crumpled position. The door creaked and groaned as I forced the bent hinges to yield, and it opened. Bending low, I looked into the tiny car and was amazed by the size of the man lying across the seats. He was big—easily more than six feet tall and at least three hundred pounds. "Why would such a huge man drive such a little car?" my brain wondered irrationally. I had watched enough TV to know about car accidents and that I should not move the victim, but this person wasn't breathing. Reaching into the car, I grabbed his left arm and pulled. Nothing. His arm gave limply to my pulling, but his body didn't move an inch. He was wedged tightly between the seats and the dashboard.

"I wouldn't do that if I were you." A slow country drawl heralded the arrival of the man in plaid.

"He's not breathing," I said. "We need to start CPR. Help me get him out."

The man in plaid leaned down and looked in the car. A look of disgust wrinkled his sun-aged face. "Not me!" he said as he turned away. "I'm not going to get sued." Shock and anger filled me. This was the high plains of New Mexico, where everyone was a neighbor!

Turning my back to the man in plaid to watch in silent witness, I gained new strength from my anger and managed to get the dying man's huge legs pried out from under the dash. He was wearing sandals, and one flew back behind me as I grabbed a leg on either side. Heaving my body backward, I pulled as hard as I could. My own sandals that I had cursed while running through the tumbleweeds slipped in the soft New Mexico dust, sending me hard to the ground. My jeans ripped on the door as I fell, and I felt the strength gained from my moment of anger drain away. I wanted to cry.

A gentle hand on my shoulder startled me out of the chaos that filled my mind. "Hi. My name is Brian. I'm an EMT. Can I help?" A flood of relief flashed through me at the recognition that here was a person with not only the will to help but the training to do so.

I couldn't explain fast enough. "He's not breathing, and I can't find a pulse, and no one will help me get him out of the car," I gasped from my position on the ground. "And that man doesn't want to get sued," I added, glaring at the man in the plaid shirt who still stood as witness.

Brian's calm face turned toward my companion so fearful of litigation. "I'm an EMT with the local ambulance service," he repeated, "and I'll take full responsibility. Now get over here and help." His voice was calm but firm, and the man in plaid followed his orders without question or comment.

With all three of us pulling and adjusting legs and arms, we were able to get the huge man out of his car. His face was now a grayish-blue color, and the frothy sputum had been replaced with the remains of whatever breakfast he had consumed that morning. Brian bent over him and scooped the vomit out of the way with his hands. Pinching the man's nostrils, he placed his mouth over the man's and gave him two breaths. "Do you know CPR?" he asked as he casually swept more vomit away.

My eyes were fixed on the big man's blue face as my lips spoke the first thing my brain thought. "I took the class six years ago, but I've let my card expire."

Brian paused in his efforts. His face turned toward me, and his eyes held mine. In all of this madness, his eyes were calm, and little smile lines folded at their corners as he spoke. "That's O.K.," he said. "I won't tell if you won't. Do it anyway."

The training came back easily as I found the proper hand position and began doing compressions on the dying man's chest. Bone crunched and time blurred. My shoulders and back ached. I was aware of the smell of vomit and blood, the oozing gray slime that protruded past the man's hair and through the crack in his skull with every compression, and the sound of the ambulance sirens.

Another hand fell on my shoulder. "Hi. I'm Rob. I'll take over now."

I forgot my paper at the store. I drove home and stood in the driveway. It all looked the same. Nothing here had changed. The grass still rustled in the breeze, my porch swing keeping time to some unknown rhythm. Sun glinted off the windows where my children slept. I took it all in, and then I cried. I cried for the man who died; I cried for the man in the plaid shirt who wouldn't help. I cried for the people in the truck and all the people who stood and watched. I cried for my torn jeans and scratched feet. I cried for the frustration of not being able to help. I cried for the cattle that would get on the highway now that the fence was down. I sat on my porch swing rocking in the breeze, and I cried.

Brian called the next day. He had tracked down my phone number through Gina at the store. Still calm and reassuring, he asked if I was O.K., adding that some of the calls still bothered him. He said he was impressed at my performance (CPR-card comment aside) and asked if I had ever considered being an EMT.

Thus began my life in and dedication to the world of emergency medical service or EMS. I became a volunteer firefighter, EMT, paramedic, and registered nurse, and taught others to do the same. I no longer live in the high plains of New Mexico. My children are grown, and even though I keep planning to buy a new one, I no longer have a porch swing. But I still have my morning coffee with my Sunday paper before the world wakes up.

Thanks, Brian, wherever you are. We all wonder sometimes if we make a difference. You did.

REASONS

Everything happens for a reason. I suppose that is part of faith, believing that pain has a purpose and that the proverbial silver lining is always shining through. The most iconic individuals in my life have held to that belief and passed it on to me. I believe that the people who hold to that belief are the ones who can take tragedy and pain and turn it into life lessons. They build over the crumpling foundations with added strength and renew their design of life.

I never knew who the man in the car was who died on the highway in New Mexico on that summer morning, but I do know and appreciate the changes he made in me and my perception of priorities. I found out later through the local paper that he had a history of heart problems and had been having chest pains for several days. He had called friends and told them he was going to drive over to the clinic and get checked out. The paper said that the people in the truck that hit him claimed he never slowed down and never even looked up; his car just flew up in front of them. His autopsy showed that he'd died of a massive heart attack. Speculation was that he died while driving and was probably dead when his car went onto the highway—before he was struck broadside by the pickup.

His death created in me a need to understand the life process. I was always fascinated with medicine. Now I needed to know how the heart worked and how it could just stop while someone was driving down the road. The more I studied, the more I became amazed with the miracles that exist within us to keep us alive every second of every day.

I never again met the man in the plaid shirt and am not sure that I would recognize him if I did. I acknowledge his contribution to the cathartic events of that tragedy. He uncovered in me the need to help others partly because he wouldn't. In time, I realized that it probably wasn't that he was truly afraid of being sued. It's not that he, or the others with him, wouldn't help but rather that some simply cannot. Facing trauma and blood is a difficult task; looking death in the face is simply impossible for some. He did what he was capable of. I hope, somehow, he learned from it.

For me it started a new path that led to some incredible places.

"DON'T TELL MOMMA!"

P arked on the corner waiting for clearance to go in, we had been dispatched to a shooting. Violence was not unusual, especially in the area of this city that was known for the turf wars between the different gangs. It had taken us three minutes to get here from our quarters, with flashing red lights and sirens screaming. A fast response, and we were in limbo, parked behind the fire engine for fifteen minutes waiting for the police department to make sure it was safe enough for us to go in. We had already been told via the radio that we had one male patient in his midthirties with a gunshot wound to the leg. Our adrenaline had started to wane after the wait and the fact that it probably wasn't a life-threatening injury. My mind turned to the coming weekend, and my partner turned the FM onto some rock and roll at a low level. We continued to wait.

"Medic three, scene cleared by PD. Approach, code two. Engine fifteen cancelled." This was confirmation that the injury was non-life-threatening. Dispatchers would never cancel the engine if they thought we were going to need the manpower it provided.

My partner put the ambulance into drive, and I confirmed with the dispatcher that we had heard her instructions. The engine fired up, and we waved good-bye to the firefighters as we pulled up around the corner to the scene that waited for us.

Easy to spot with three police cars nosed into the sidewalk, our patient sat quietly on the curb with his leg extended in front of him surrounded by police officers. He was a big man. Although it was hard to judge from the way he was leaning forward, I could tell he was well over six feet tall. Big and very muscular through the shoulders, he looked as though, given different circumstances, he could have been a professional football player. As it was, he sat slumped on the curb, his gang colors lying on the sidewalk next to him.

I opened my door as one of the police sergeants approached to give me the run down. "Looks like we've got some gang stuff coming down," he said. "Vic's name is Jared. Says he and his buds were 'just hanging out,' and someone shot into the group of them for no reason." The expected smirk traveled across his face fleetingly. If you listened to the stories of the people who ended up on the wrong side of the law, it was never their own doing that got them into trouble. They were always "just standing here minding my own business" when someone or something did something bad to them. "One of these days," he continued, "these gangbangers are going to learn to aim when they do their drive-by shootings, and then we'll all be really busy."

I walked next to him and back around to the side of the ambulance where the huge wounded man, sans his gang-colored shirt, sat waiting with his head down. "He's not very communicative, but we've had a history going back to his high-school-dropout days. Hadn't seen him around for a while. Thought he had managed to get out. Come on, Jared," he said to the guy on the ground. "Time to get up. Your ride is here."

Jared never looked up but pulled his uninjured leg under him and stretched to his full height. He was easily six foot five, and I knew this ride was not going to be comfortable for him as ambulance gurneys were not designed to hold anyone over about five foot ten comfortably. Jared hopped over to the back of the rig and, with my partner's assistance, managed to pull himself up and swing around to the gurney. He had to sit with his good knee folded and his left leg extended over the side and up onto the bench seat. I jumped in behind him and, stepping carefully over his injured leg, proceeded with my medical assessment.

He had a single gunshot wound to the lower leg with an entrance and exit wound. There was only a slow ooze of blood coming from the wounds, definitely not life threatening. "How far away was the shooter?" I asked Jared. No response. He just kept staring down at his hands. I put sterile dressings over the wounds and pulled out my blood-pressure cuff. "Jared, I know this is traumatic for you, but you are going to have to answer some questions here in a minute." I gave him warning before my paperwork and the barrage of questions that would come with it. Lifting his arm to take his blood pressure, I had to switch to the thigh cuff in order to reach all the way around his huge bicep. Thinking that the musculature in his exposed chest and arms was due to steroids, I asked first, "Are you taking any medications or supplements?" No answer. As complacent as Jared was, he was not going to be easy to get any answers from.

The sergeant was still standing at the rear doors. "Come on, Jared. The lady is just trying to help," he said, shaking his head as he closed the doors.

Glancing in the rearview mirror to make sure I was set, my partner started the engine, and we headed for the county hospital. The sergeant pulled his cruiser in behind us and followed. I guessed he wasn't quite done with Jared.

"Are you allergic to any medications?" No answer. "Jared, do you have any medical problems that I need to know about?" Still no answer. "O.K., Jared, we can do it your way. But you're going to have to answer questions when we get to the hospital." I sighed. I did not want to fight with this big guy.

"Jared, is there someone we can call to meet you at the hospital? Would that make it easier?" I tried once more and pulled back in surprise when Jared's shoulders started to shake, slowly at first.

"Jared, are you O.K.?" I said, placing a hand on his big shoulder. It started to shake harder, and I became more concerned. This guy could squish me with one hand. "Jared?" Suddenly great sobs escaped from Jared, in addition to his now violently heaving shoulders. This huge gang-member giant was crying! I placed my hand on his shoulder. "Aw, Jared. What can I do?" I asked.

And then, staggered in between giant sobbing breaths, Jared finally spoke. "Please," he gasped. "Please...don't...tell...my...momma!"

I pulled back against the bench seat and surveyed this huge, sobbing giant. "What?" It wasn't my most eloquent question, but it was all I could manage.

Now Jared looked up at me. With huge tears running down his cheeks and sobs racking his chest, he repeated his plea. "Please...don't...tell...my...momma...She goin' to...kill...me!"

I stared in amazement. I had been working this area for years and thought I had seen everything. But this was different. "Jared, you're a grown man. I'm not going to tell anyone you don't want to know about this," I reassured him, stroking his giant, quaking shoulder as one does a nervous horse.

"You...don'...understand," he continued. "She goin'...to kill...me!" He gasped out the last and buried his giant face in his huge hands as the sobs continued to shake him and the gurney.

I did not know where to go with this. My eyes met my partner's in the rearview mirror. I saw the concern in his eyes and shrugged my shoulders in answer to his question. I had no idea how to handle this one.

It was a ten-minute transport to the county hospital, and Jared sobbed the whole way. As the ambulance swung wide and started to back in, I counseled him on controlling his sobs so we could safely unload the gurney. He was a big man and hung over the sides of the bed, which in itself created some hazards. "Deep breaths, Jared. Try to stay calm." He took deep, gasping sighs of air but controlled his shuddering as we unloaded the gurney with him on it. My partner lifted the foot end, arching back to avoid the injured leg, and I lowered the legs of the gurney to the pavement. Straightening back up, I saw Jared's eyes go as wide as saucers. The color drained from his face as panic consumed it. Whirling about in fear and remembering that this was a gang shooting, I was met with the sight of a diminutive little woman. She could not have been more than five feet tall or weighed more than ninety pounds dripping wet. She had graying hair pulled back in a bun that hovered over the starched collar of her flowered housedress, and clutched up against her ample bosom, she held a double-handled handbag of shiny tan pleather. She was the only other person in the ambulance bay, and I relaxed a little. However, Jared again began to shudder and sob. That's when Momma came to life. Walking over to the side of the gurney, she reached up with her bag and—*whack*—smacked Jared across the head.

"No…Momma!" wailed Jared. *Whack, whack* went the pleather purse. Jared covered his head with his hands, and Momma wailed away at him.

"I done tol' you to stay away from that crowd!" yelled Momma. "You got a wife and a boy to be lookin' after!" *Whack, whack* went the purse.

"No, Momma, no!" yelled Jared.

My partner and I took either end of the gurney, avoiding Momma as best we could. Entering the code into the ambulance-bay keypad, we wheeled in Jared with little Momma following right along and whacking him whenever she could reach high enough to hit him.

The sergeant, who had arrived at the same time that we did, chuckled as he walked up. "I see you've met Momma." He grinned.

Wheeling the gurney into the assigned room, we assisted Jared onto the hospital bed and lowered it. Momma appreciated that because it was not nearly as high as our gurney and her five-foot reach was much more effective. *Whack, whack.* "No, Momma, no!" And the sergeant chuckled.

Somehow, I think I know who told Momma.

"LONG WAY TO GO"

I was working in the hills that day. One of the pleasures of working twenty-four-hour shifts was the ability to increase the household income by picking up per-diem jobs in other locations. This was a small, three-ambulance company that provided service for one of the counties located up in the foothills. It was a good change of pace from my usual city runs.

The fall air was crisp with winter, but the summer sun still lingered in the afternoons, which was a nice break from the previous week of rain and snow that had soaked the roads and made traveling difficult.

I was working with a new partner, Sam. He had lived in the area for years, and from what I had heard from the other medics I worked with, he was a good EMT. The station was a two-bedroom trailer tucked under some pine trees in a little town that could brag about a gas station but still didn't have any traffic lights. The serenity of the setting was therapeutic, and sometimes I would pull the extra shifts just to sit under those trees for a few hours and listen to the wind dance through the branches. The volume of calls was low because people in these small towns just didn't call for an ambulance unless it was truly an emergency.

The morning passed by slowly as it always did in this area. This was what the people in the valley referred to as one of the vacation stations: nice quarters, quiet area, and not a lot of calls. In exchange, a responder up here had to accept that the intensity of the calls could be dramatic, with longer response times to the call locations and a corresponding length of transport times to the hospitals.

We worked primarily with volunteer firefighters up here. The volunteers were a very dedicated breed, responding to calls on their own time and without remuneration. Training was intense for these loyal community members, and I was constantly amazed at the longevity of the locals' commitment to their neighbors.

We had finished checking the rig out early. The rest of the morning and afternoon were, in fact, like a vacation. I had visited with Sam for a while, finished a novel that I had been carrying with me, walked around the park, eaten a leisurely lunch, and even taken a nap. We had no calls, and I was really enjoying the pace.

Sam and I were kicking back in the lounge chairs watching some TV. It had started to snow gently outside, and I was considering an early bedtime. It was only around 8:00 p.m., but the pace was relaxing, and the fall air was perfect for sleeping. I was just extricating myself from the recliner to move to my bedroom when the phone rang. This area was dispatched by phone due to the difficulties with radios in the mountains, but relaxation had taken over. I was surprised when Sam said, "We've got a call out at the Point."

The Point was another community farther up in the hills. It was known as a tough town. Its inhabitants lived there, for the most part, because they didn't like people. They carried guns and were known for their vigilante ways. It had been originally populated in the gold-rush days, and the taste of the Wild West occasionally still lingered. It would take us twenty to thirty minutes to arrive, but the Point's volunteer fire department should have been able to get there in about ten minutes. The call was for "difficulty breathing in a patient with asthma."

I let the relaxation that had taken over continue as Sam drove the ambulance with lights and siren through the canyon that separated our station from the outlying town. We had already done a prealert to the hospital telling them that we were responding to an asthma patient with a thirty-minute-to-on-scene time. Sam and I chatted about the area and the type of people who called it home intermittently as we listened to the scanner in the ambulance. The snow continued to fall, and a light dusting covered the pines.

The fire department, as expected, had arrived at the patient's house within ten to fifteen minutes. We were still about five minutes out when the radio spoke again. "Notify the medics that we've got CPR in progress."

The relaxation left in a hurry as I questioned Sam about what I already knew I had heard. "Did they say what I think they said?" Sam nodded his head and asked me how I wanted the code run. Every muscle was now wide awake as I quickly covered my outline for running a full arrest with Sam. I trusted Sam but had never before run a full code with him. "I'll have a quick look while you set up my tubes. Nothing smaller than number seven. I'll tell you after I see the patient what size. While I'm tubing, you get the line set up and pull my first line of drugs. Have the fire department get the backboard for us while we're doing that. Anything else we'll do on the way to the hospital."

Sam glanced over at me. "In this weather it will take around forty-five minutes to get to the hospital, you know."

I did know. I wasn't looking forward to it. I quickly updated the hospital as we pulled around the last bend in the road and started looking for the right address. Not all of the houses up there were marked, and sometimes it was difficult to find them. Luckily the fire departments that worked these areas were usually thoughtful enough to leave a bright-orange cone marker at the driveway.

Up ahead we saw a large man waving us down at the bottom of a steep driveway marked with the orange cone. The snowflakes were larger, and the rate of their descent had become more aggressive as if the skies had felt the end of the vacation period too. Sam said, "Looks like they left one of the firefighters with the marker cone this time. Poor guy standing in the snow." We pulled up next to the man, and

Sam rolled his window down. "Jump in," Sam said to the man. "We'll give you a ride up. Sounds like we're going to need all the help we can get."

The man jumped in the back of the ambulance and sat down in the jump seat directly behind the driver's compartment. "Driveway's pretty bad. And it's a long one." He said, "You got four-wheel drive in this thing?" Sam assured him that we did, and we proceeded up toward the house.

The driveway was steep and muddy. The rear of the ambulance swung back and forth as Sam pushed it up the hill. Looking out the side window, I saw the steep drop-off to the bottom of the canyon. In order to distract myself from the driveway, I introduced myself to the man and asked him if he had any update. A confused look crossed his face as he asked me what I meant by update. "New firefighter," I thought to myself. "He doesn't know the lingo yet."

"I mean, do you know what's going on?" I said.

The man took the rain- and snow-soaked hat from his head and ran his hand through his hair. "Yeah," he said, "the wife's got asthma, and she's been having trouble all day. I finally talked her into letting me call you people."

With horror I realized that this man, whom I assumed was a firefighter, was the patient's husband and that he had no idea what was going on in his own home. I turned and looked out the window again. The steep drop-off into the bottomless canyon was now my distraction.

Sam spoke up. "You been waiting down there long?" The man explained that after he had talked his wife into letting him call 911, he had walked to the bottom of the driveway and waited for us.

The rear end of the ambulance again slid in a wide arch as we topped the incline and the house came into sight. "Sir." I broke the silence. "Our last report from the fire department said your wife is not doing very well. I didn't want you to go into the house without knowing that."

Jumping out of the rig, I grabbed my respiratory bag and the cardiac monitor. The patient's husband was already going up the steps to the house, and I followed him in. Sam was right behind me with the drug box when the man from the driveway froze in his tracks at the bedroom door. "God damn it!" he screamed as he turned and punched a hole in the bedroom door with his fist with the ease of a knife slicing through butter. "God damn it!" he screamed again as he punched another hole, sending wood splinters flying in all directions. One of the firefighters gently took the man's shoulder and tried to lead him out of the doorway, allowing me to slip into the room.

There on the floor was the man's wife. One firefighter was forcing air into her lungs with a bag-valve mask while another did chest compressions. I dropped to my knees and grabbed for my cardiac monitor. "How long?" I asked.

The female firefighter who was doing the chest compressions looked up at me. "She dropped right after we got here about ten minutes ago. We started CPR right away."

My cardiac monitor showed an asystolic rhythm, a flat line. "Hyperventilate her!" I said as I moved to the woman's head and prepared to insert a tube that would hold her airway open. I slipped through the vocal cords easily on the first try. Quickly securing it in place, I attached the bag-valve mask to the tube. Pulling my stethoscope from around my neck, I listened to the woman's chest. The sound of her lungs was faint and filled with wheezes and rhonchi, but it was there as the firefighter continued to push air into her lungs. I glanced up at the monitor. There were a few wide beats showing now. Our patient had obviously gone down from a lack of oxygen. The tightness of her lungs had prohibited the oxygen from getting to her heart, and it had slowed down until it had stopped. Forcing the air back into her lungs was giving life back to her heart.

"Sam, give me the epi," I said. "We're going down the tube with it." Sam had the drug I had requested in my hand and ready to go before I had even finished the sentence. He was good.

The mechanism that secured the airway tube and the drug, which hopefully would excite the heart and assist in dilating the lungs, were in place. I moved down to the woman's arm and started an IV as fast as I could.

I listened again to the woman's lungs. Still tight. I needed to do more to open them. Pushing another epi down the tube, I told Sam to set me up a Proventil TX and get the stuff together to rig it to the tube. I wanted to call the hospital now and let them know what we were dealing with.

Unable to reach the hospital on the radio, I grabbed a phone off the woman's bedside table. The nurse that answered was short and rude when I dismissed her and asked for the doctor. Time was of the essence here. I was telling the doctor what I was doing when I heard a loud thump coming from the living room. Glancing up, I was horrified to see one of the volunteer firefighters fly into the room backward and crash into the wall opposite the bedroom door. He immediately came to his feet and slammed the door shut. "They've gone crazy," he yelled. "The family has gone crazy!" He had the door wedged shut with his body, but we could hear the enraged family pounding on it. Sam jumped to his feet and helped push the door shut to lock it.

I grabbed my radio and threw it to Sam. "Get SO up here. We don't have time for this."

The doctor was still talking. I asked him to repeat his orders, explaining that we were having some trouble with the family. He concurred that the treatment I wanted was appropriate for this patient. Unfortunately, I would never have time to administer all of it.

My EKG monitor showed that the patient's heart was responding to the drugs we had given. I reached down and felt for a pulse. Yes! She had a pulse. It was weak, but her heart was working with us. I asked one of the firefighters to get me a blood pressure and moved around to administer the drug that the doctor had ordered.

"You had better look at this." The female firefighter had a look of deep concern on her face as she spoke. "This isn't right."

Leaving the drug where I was working, I moved over to the patient. Her neck was swelling up, and with a gentle touch I felt air under her skin. My own pulse increased dramatically as I recognized the condition known as subcutaneous emphysema. The feel and sound of it are not unlike rubbing your hands on Saran wrap, and it is not a good sign. I listened again to her lungs. On the left, I heard good air movement; on the right...nothing.

The angry sounds of the family were still on the other side of the door as I moved back to the telephone. The doctor answered this time as I told him that I was going to have to decompress the chest. I also quickly explained that we were currently locked in the bedroom but that the sheriff's office was on its way. I had never done a chest decompression in the field before and asked the doctor to guide me through it. The procedure consists of inserting a large needle into the chest to relieve air pressure from the cavity between the lung and the chest wall. When air gets into this cavity from either a hole in the chest wall or a hole in the lung itself, it causes the lung to collapse. This is what was happening to our patient. Inserting the needle in the chest either through a site below the clavicle bone or on the patient's side would hopefully allow the air inside to come out and let the lung reinflate.

The doctor was running through the procedure we had studied in school so diligently. As he spoke, I was watching the woman's chest blow up like a balloon. He was telling me to decompress from the subclavicular area, which is the site close between the patient's throat and shoulder. I stopped the doctor in midsentence. "Doc, she has no subclavicular landmarks available. The sub-Q has blown up her chest. I'm going in through the midaxillary site." All the in-class practice paid off as the training took over and the fear left.

Reaching for the supplies I needed, I was interrupted by Sam. "Connie, SO can't make it. All their cars are busy. CHP is on the way, but they don't have a four-wheel drive in the area."

"Deal with it," I snapped. This was nuts.

Air flowed out with a hissing sound from the newly inserted needle in the patient's chest as I again listened to her chest. The procedure had worked. Both lungs were inflating with every squeeze of the life-giving oxygen bag.

"Uh, Connie." It was the female firefighter again. "She's in V-fib." I whirled around and looked at my monitor. What else could happen? Grabbing the paddles of my EKG monitor, I sent two-hundred joules of electricity through the woman's body. She jerked slightly as the electricity went through. I watched the monitor. Her heart was working with us again—nice, normal sinus rhythm. I reached for a preload of lidocaine, a drug used to stop the heart from getting too excited.

As I was inserting the drug into the IV, Sam spoke again. "CHP is at the bottom of the driveway. They don't have a four-wheel drive available and can't get their cars up the hill."

I took a deep breath and pulled back for a minute. Surveying the scene was unreal. This woman had been alive and fine this afternoon. Now here we were fighting her body for her life, trapped in her bedroom, with her family beating on the door outside. Suddenly I was angry—very angry. Without a word I stood up and went to the door.

Sam stepped aside but voiced his concern. "What are you doing? They're hitting people, and I know they've got guns."

I ignored them all. I had had it. One battle at a time was enough, and the fight with death took priority.

Irrational because of my anger, I pushed through the door and walked right into the husband's chest. My normally calm composure was gone as I confronted him. "What the hell do you think you are doing?" I screamed at him, jabbing my finger into his broad chest. "I am trying to save her life. She keeps coming and going! She needs a hospital, and I can't get her there because you are all being stupid!" The man's face hung as he looked in astonishment at this little female paramedic who was obviously more out of control then he was.

"Calm down, miss." Suddenly he was the one who wanted the situation to be more rational. "We didn't expect her to die is all. What do you want me to do?"

I was shaking from anger and frustration as I stuck my finger into his chest yet again. "I want you to get your family the hell out of my way so that I can try to save your wife's life!" With that I turned and went back into the bedroom.

The two firefighters by the door had the same look of shock on their faces as the woman's husband. "What do you want us to do?" one of them asked.

I was on a roll. "I want you to get my gurney and get this lady to my ambulance, *now!*" Everyone parted as I made my way back to the side of my patient. She was no longer recognizable. Her heart was still fighting, but the air under her skin was so pronounced that her face was distorting. The lids of her eyes looked as if she had golf balls under them. Her appearance took the anger away from me. I rechecked her lungs and her pulses and then helped the firefighters load her into the ambulance for the trip to the hospital. The family had locked one of the patient's sons in a car somewhere to keep him out of our way, and we could hear him screaming as we rolled past.

Only the female firefighter was able to go to the hospital, and I needed two assistants. I asked Sam to get on the radio and have one of the other volunteer departments meet us halfway. At that point, the patient was holding her own, but things did not look good. Her skin seemed to blow up more and more with every breath we gave her.

I put the female firefighter in charge of breathing for the patient, and we started down the driveway. Taking a deep breath, I was assessing the situation when I heard Sam's voice. "Connie, if you don't have a seat belt on, you'd better hold on." His voice betrayed the gravity of the situation as I looked up through the front windshield. The ambulance was in a downhill slide, and there was a large pine tree right in our path. Gripping the side of the gurney, I lowered myself to the floor and braced against the patient. I held the tube going to her lungs with one hand and told the firefighter to hold on. At the last second, the ambulance found its footing, and we were back on track.

"Are all of your calls like this?" The female firefighter had a quizzical look on her face.

"God, I hope not," was my response.

My patient was blowing up like a balloon. Her heart was slowing down again. The first needle that I had inserted in her chest had been pushed out by the air under her skin and was dripping fluid. I checked her lungs and found no breath sounds on the right side. Pulling a larger needle from the shelf, I again decompressed her chest. The whistle of air through the needle did nothing to relieve the tension.

A CHP officer had fallen in behind us and was swerving his car back and forth to keep the family from passing him and catching the ambulance. He managed to stop the car behind him temporarily as we paused to pick up another volunteer for extra manpower. The firefighter had been waiting at the side of the road and jumped in even before the ambulance stopped completely. "Go," he yelled to Sam. Then he froze. His eyes got big as he stared in disbelief at my patient. The woman who had weighed 150 pounds on-scene now looked as if she weighed more than 300. "What the—?"

I didn't give him time to finish his sentence. We had been driving for fifteen minutes, and the first firefighter was getting cramps in her hands from compressing the bag-valve device. I put the new firefighter in charge of the airway and got on the radio to update the hospital. The doctor answered again. I updated him and asked if there was anything that could be done for the air under the skin. He started telling us that the subcutaneous emphysema could look dramatic, but it wasn't really a problem. Cutting him off, I told him he was going to have to see this one to believe it. I also made sure that the hospital was aware of the problem with the family and would have the city police standing by.

My mind was numb as I watched the cardiac monitor. The air under the woman's skin was making it impossible for the monitor to adequately pick up the electrical rhythm of her heart. I watched as the lines that represented the beats got smaller and smaller until they no longer showed at all. We couldn't feel a pulse anymore. The amount of air under the patient's skin was incredible. She now looked as if she weighed close to four-hundred pounds. Her fingers and toes were swollen into squash-shaped appendages. Her face was without recognizable landmarks. I felt drained.

As we pulled into the hospital parking lot, my patient's skin color began to look bad again with blue tinges forming on her lips. There was nothing more I could do. I couldn't hear breath sounds on either side, and I had no idea if she had a pulse or not due to the grotesque swelling. The doctor met us at the back door. He froze in his tracks the same way the firefighter had. "Oh my God," he said. "You didn't tell me it was this bad." Yeah, well, I tried, doc.

The patient was pronounced dead shortly thereafter. There was nothing more anyone could do for her. I finished my paperwork and was leaving the hospital when I almost ran into the son. I was too tired to try to avoid him. He looked me in the eyes and then dropped his head. "I'm sorry," he mumbled.

It wasn't his fault. None of us know how we are going to react to things until they happen. I offered him a shoulder to cry on. "I'm sorry too," I whispered. "I tried."

My eyes filled with tears as I watched him walk off. Sometimes life isn't fair. Sometimes anger is easier than grief.

GRIEF

Professionally, we are taught that there are five stages of grieving following a death or other loss: denial, bargaining, depression, anger, and finally acceptance. Usually these stages are spread out over time while the people who are feeling them attempt to assimilate the reality of the situation. The stages have no set order, and people can fluctuate between the different stages while the healing process progresses.

Most professionals have seen the dysfunctional side of these five stages of grieving, as in the previous story. Just as people do not know how they will react in any given scenario until that situation has occurred, most have no idea how they will behave in the grieving process until the unfortunate has occurred. Of all the emotions involved in these situations, I believe that anger is the easiest to rush to when it is an unexpected death. It allows for the natural adrenaline released in a fight-or-flight situation to be expressed, whereas the other four steps and the emotions that correspond with them do not.

There is a very delicate balance between allowing for expressions of grief and being trapped in unsafe situations. The family in this story reacted in a very violent manner. They endangered the first responders and themselves with their overtly physical displays of anger at their grief. Fortunately for them, this event occurred in a small community where law enforcement has the power to let things go. I was approached after this call by law enforcement wanting to know if we wished to press charges. None of us did because we have all seen it before, and while it can be dangerous, it is an honest expression of grief.

"A LESSON IN CHILDBIRTH"

Jimmy was my partner that day. He was new to the field of EMS. Jim had a look of innocence on his face that made him seem even younger than his twenty-three years. Chubby cheeks and slack jaw—he watched everything with his eyes held wide open. He had a look that could best be described as cherubic, and he was new enough to the field that he had not learned to disguise his emotions beneath the unwavering calmness required by the profession. He still wore those emotions on his sleeve for the world to see.

It was a fall morning. The air was crisp as we spent the first available hours doing our daily chores. We finished making sure that the equipment was in order and we were well stocked. The sun and cool air were enjoyable as we washed the ambulance in preparation for another shift.

Ambulance stations are all equipped with alert tones that flash lights inside the building and have speakers in the driveway to make sure the calls are heard by the people assigned to the response. Our outdoor speakers clicked on, and the tones blasted the introduction for the first call of the shift. "Medic seventy-two, respond for a woman in labor. Fifth child. Water has broken." Taking time only to shut off the water, we hopped in our freshly cleaned rig, hit the garage-door button, and responded to the call with lights and sirens.

Labor calls were very common in Stockton—especially since the recent arrival of Southeast Asian refugees. Acclimating tens of thousands of third-world people to modern culture was a difficult task. Unfortunately, many of them ended up being thrown into huge, dilapidated apartment complexes tucked away from the mainstream. They were given food stamps, welfare, and Medi-Cal and told that if they had any problems, to just dial 911. This labor call was in one of those complexes.

Southeast Asian women for the most part have an easy time with childbirth. It was very common to go on scene to one of the complexes only to be told in broken English to "Hurry! Baby come quick." It had become so common in fact that this was the slang given to these calls: baby-come-quick calls. And they usually did come quick. In fact, I quit counting the number of babies I delivered after my first year as a paramedic simply because the volume was so high.

Jimmy and I arrived with the fire department personnel to find the familiar scenario: a dilapidated apartment with mattresses lining the walls in the living room. Sitting on one of these was our mother to be, waving her Medi-Cal card in her hand. Very rarely did anyone, including the mother, speak any English. We had a ten-year-old boy, the only English-speaking person in the apartment, translate the most necessary of the information. We needed to know a due date, number of babies living, number of pregnancies, which doctor, and which hospital. The length and duration of the contractions would have to be determined in the back of the ambulance with a gentle hand on the mother's stomach. In such a strict societal structure, asking personal questions of a ten year old would embarrass everyone. We knew that the amniotic sack had already ruptured because of the wet sarong and the warm, musky smell that permeated the living room. The small woman was moved to the gurney and then to the ambulance.

Normally these calls would be handed off to the EMT partner, since in our county a baby-come-quick call was Basic Life Support skill until after the baby was delivered. Jim, however, seemed very nervous about the call. He placed himself at the foot of the gurney and had his gloves off his hands before anyone else. Making a mental note to talk to Jimmy in private later, I jumped in the back with our patient, waved good-bye to the fire department, and told Jimmy what to say on the radio when he called it in to the hospital.

This woman, like most in her community, was the patient of Dr. Phong and was going to the hospital at which he primarily practiced. Dr. Phong was himself of Southeast Asian heritage. A small man with a huge smile and a quick wit, Dr. Phong was a top-notch OB.

En route to the hospital, I did the standard care. I checked my patient's blood pressure, pulse rate, and respiratory rate. Next, I placed my hand on the woman's belly with a reassuring smile so that my non-English-speaking patient would not feel her territory invaded. Her distended belly tightened under my hand, and I glanced at my watch...fifteen seconds...thirty seconds...forty seconds...good contraction. I removed my hand and reached for my pen to jot down a few notes. I had barely copied the patient's name from her card to my prehospital form when I noticed a slight grimace on her face. Contractions less than a minute apart!

Making eye contact with my patient, I mimed the breathing pattern I wanted her to follow, which would keep her from pushing. "Blow, blow, blow." I coached her through the contraction.

"Jimmy, tell the hospital that this one is close. We may deliver before we get there," I called to my partner, while reaching up for an obstetrical kit. The OB kit contained everything needed for an emergency childbirth.

I pulled the patient's sarong up to her thighs. The baby's head was not yet visible, but the area surrounding the birth canal was pushed out in preparation for the baby's arrival. This one would be close.

We arrived at the hospital and quickly pulled the gurney from the back of the ambulance. Our pace was much faster than normal— mine because I didn't want to deliver yet another baby in the lobby of the hospital or in the elevator. Jimmy, however, looked frightened, almost panicked. "Jimmy, have you never delivered a baby?" I asked as we rode up in the elevator.

Jimmy's eyes fell to the floor, and he flushed from the neck up. "No," he replied, "I've never even seen a baby being born. I was kind of hoping this one would come so I could watch you deliver it."

The doors to the elevator opened, and we resumed our quick pace to the OB ward. Dr. Phong met us at the entrance. Looking at me with his quick smile and intense eyes, he asked in the lingo of EMS, "Baby come quick?"

I laughed and assured him that this baby was going to make his or her entrance into the world without delay. "Dr. Phong," I asked, "my partner has never seen a child birth. Would you mind if he watched?"

Jimmy blushed full in the face this time, looking down at the floor. "Oh no," he stammered. "That's O.K."

Dr. Phong chuckled at Jimmy's response. "Best to learn baby delivery from the best." He grabbed my partner by the arm and steered him into the delivery room with our patient. Addressing her in her own language, he gestured toward Jimmy and laughed. The patient smiled shyly at Jimmy and nodded an affirmation to Dr. Phong's question. Dr. Phong turned to face Jimmy. "She say O.K.," he said in his thick accent. "You want to watch baby come? I do better than that. You going to deliver the baby!"

This time Jimmy turned white. Those huge eyes grew even bigger as horror filled his face. "No, no!" He was almost begging now as he said, "That's O.K., really," as he tried to back out of the room.

Dr. Phong was too quick for him though. Grabbing Jimmy's arm, he pushed him back toward our patient, who was now draped and gowned by the efficient OB nurses. "No," Dr. Phong said, "you going to learn to deliver my patients' babies from best baby doctor in town."

I smiled. Most of our patients who delivered in the ambulance were indeed Dr. Phong's patients. Jimmy was still protesting as Dr. Phong forced him over to our patient. Her legs were now propped up in the stirrups and spread wide in preparation for the birth of her baby. Dr. Phong grabbed Jimmy by the shoulders and turned him to face the little woman. When Jimmy saw the patient's presentation, he froze in his tracks and was struck mute in his protestations. His face was whiter than the sheet that draped our patient, and his jaw dropped open. "Close mouth," Dr. Phong laughed. "You going to catch flies!"

By now I was laughing out loud along with our patient. The site of Jimmy's horror distracted everyone except the OB nurse who flew around the room efficiently following Dr. Phong's orders. She ripped open a package of sterile gloves and snapped one on Jimmy's right hand. The glove on his hand broke Jimmy's trance as his eyes fell from the patient to the nurse who was approaching with the left glove. "No, no," Jimmy mumbled. "I don't need two—"

Dr. Phong now joined the patient and me in our laughter. He was thoroughly enjoying his new pupil. "Oh," he said in mock seriousness, "you much better than me then. You catch with one hand?"

The serious little nurse now joined in the laughter as she snapped the other glove on Jimmy's left hand. Our patient however had become quiet, and turning to look at her, we all noticed a slight grimace on her face.

Dr. Phong was in his moment. Grabbing Jimmy by the arm again and steering him even closer to the patient, he cried, "There! You see that?" He gestured toward the patient's face. "Southeast Asian women not feel pain. Patient make this face..." And Dr. Phong screwed his face into a perfect replica of our patient's grimace. "She going to have baby now."

Jimmy hadn't laughed once in all of this. He stood with his eyes wide open as his gaze fell from the patient's face to the area from which the baby would soon emerge. His face became stoic as he crouched in a position that I could only describe as a quarterback preparing for the hike. Jimmy stared straight ahead at the area that had become his nemesis as Dr. Phong continued his educational lecture on the sociology of childbirth.

"Now, Jimmy, that be Asian woman. If this be black woman, she be going like this..." Dr. Phong arched his back and thrust his stomach forward. He grabbed at his belly in the perfect depiction of a pregnant woman's posture. Rolling his body from side to side, his Southeast Asian accent instantly vanished as he spoke fluent Ebonics. "Hep me, hep me, oh lordy, hep me!" he cried, "I's dyin'." I held my stomach too with laughter as Dr. Phong continued. "White woman *meeean* when she have baby. When she get to this point, she grab husband like this," Dr. Phong grabbed Jimmy by his shirt collar, and again his accent vanished, only this time it became the voice of an angry white woman. "'You did this to me!' she say to husband. 'You never touching me again!'"

Jimmy hadn't heard a word. Even with Dr. Phong grabbing his collar, he had stayed frozen in the crouch staring straight ahead.

The nurses from the station had also arrived at the door to the room and were in hysterics as Dr. Phong next addressed the Hispanic race. "Now if this be Mexican woman," he said, "she grab edge of bed like this, sit straight up, and just scream and scream and scream. Then she stop to pray to all the saints, then she scream again."

Jimmy let out a small squeak, and we all turned to look. The baby's head was now showing. Dr. Phong discontinued his wonderful rendition of the cultural diversity of childbirth as he directed Jimmy on what to do next. Jimmy successfully delivered the baby with Dr. Phong's help and went on to become a very good paramedic. A small son made his entrance into the world that day in a room full of laughter and good cheer. Jimmy, however, does not remember a word that was spoken.

BABIES

As an EMS provider, I was constantly quizzed on whether or not I had ever delivered a baby. There is an underlying belief that it is all glorious and miraculous. Miraculous, yes, but I definitely would not call the process itself glorious. It involves pain, fear, danger, and various body fluid discharges that present an interesting array of odors, none of which will ever be displayed in a department store lineup of desirable colognes.

I had begun my career during a period when a large population unschooled in the ways of our modern society was instructed to call 911 for pretty much anything medical—including childbirth. During my first year as a paramedic, I delivered enough babies that I lost count. Most of the deliveries were simple presentations of a new life with no complications, and I simply assisted women to whom childbirth was a natural part of life. Prior to their introduction into our mechanized society, these same women would have been assisted by a midwife in a village hut in a scenario repeated since the beginning of time.

Americans have transformed this simple act into a mystical, involved drama that takes places in a protected and sterile environment devoid of the human interaction that makes it a family affair. This very removal from the safe bounds of family and society have turned a normal process into a frightful affair for patient and family, which in turn creates a painful process for all involved. Still the introduction of a new human life into this crazy, mixed-up world has almost always been a celebration for us. There is an indescribable joy in the first angry cry of a healthy newborn being thrust into this life: a reaffirmation of the renewal of creation.

AN UNUSUAL THANK-YOU

I t was an everyday transfer. One of the local clinics was sending an elderly gentleman with chest pain to a more appropriate treating facility. There was a possibility that he was having a heart attack, and although we could get rid of the pain for him, he would need medicine that was more aggressive in order to get well.

We had put the gentleman into the back of the ambulance strapped to the gurney, and I climbed in beside him. I made sure that he was hooked up to the cardiac monitor, that the oxygen was flowing, and that his IV was all right. He assured me that he wasn't having any chest pain at the time, so we began chatting. "You people are incredible," he said. "I can't believe you do the job that you do." I thanked him. We don't hear words of appreciation much, and when we do, it means a lot.

"The first time I met a female paramedic was when my grand-daughter got hurt," he continued. "She was only three and a half years old at the time. Her sister and my daughter were doing some canning when the water fell on the baby."

My mind raced. I recognized the call. "Really," I said. "Was your granddaughter hurt badly?"

He watched out the back door of the ambulance as he continued his story. "Well, the doctors said that the paramedics saved her. They said that if the paramedics hadn't acted so fast, she could have been horribly disfigured or even died. We lived on Ash Street in Lodi at the time..."

My mind raced back. That was my call. I remembered it vividly. We were sent for "a burn victim. No additional information available." Arriving on scene, we were met at the curb by an hysterical family. The father was holding a limp multicolored quilt that he shoved at me as I stepped out the side door of the ambulance. I met my partner at the back doors and climbed in holding the little bundle. It mewed softly like a small kitten, and when I gently unwrapped it, I found a small child. There was a teenage girl standing near the opening to the back door screaming over and over, "It was my fault! It was my fault!" Leaving my partner to deal with the chaos outside, I gently unwrapped the delicate little package that had been thrust at me. Pulling the quilt away from her little body, I was horrified to see that the skin was already sloughing away. She had burns on her face, head, and the entire right side of her body. She was crying and screaming in pain and fear as I laid her on the gurney, placed sterile burn sheets over the worst areas, and started cooling the burns with bottles of sterile water we kept on the shelf for such a purpose.

My partner, who had been dealing with the craziness outside the ambulance, called to me through the back doors. "The sister is burned too. It's only on her feet. Do you want to take her or get another ambulance?" Since we were in a northern bedroom community, and the nearest burn center was twenty miles south of the metropolitan area, I told him to put her in the jump seat.

Now I had two patients, my second being the hysterical teenager. While I pulled towels and cooled the reddening wounds on the baby, my partner fastened her sister into the jump seat. Hearing her cries agitated my little patient even more. "Jill." I spoke to her more sharply than I had intended, but this was serious. "If you don't be quiet, I am going to make you wait for another ambulance. Do you hear me? Your sister is hurt badly, and I will not have you upset her. Now I need you to help me. Can you do that?"

Jill calmed down almost immediately. She looked shocked that I had spoken to her in that tone. "Jill, will you stay calm?" Jill nodded her head. "O.K., Jill, here is some sterile water and towels. I need you to help me cool off your sister's burns." She began to focus on her sister and didn't say anything. I could see why. The tears still welled in her eyes as she applied the cooling towels to her sister's head and face.

In the meantime, my partner had finished setting up the IV that I would be using on the small one. "Let's roll," I told him. "Code three."

Jill remained calm while I addressed the tot. The child was in terrible pain, and it broke my heart to see it. About all I could do was cool off the burns and give her pain medication if she would let me. "Sweetheart," I addressed her as calmly as possible, "I can give you some medicine to make the pain go away if you will let me."

I had her attention. "Will it hurt?" she whimpered, already fatigued from the pain of the burns. I couldn't lie to this baby. It was going to hurt. "Honey, do you see this little blue spot right here?" I asked her, pointing to the tiny little vein in the unburned arm. "I have to poke it with a needle one time to give you the medicine. It's going to hurt for just a minute but not nearly as badly as the other stuff hurts."

She looked at me with a question in her big blue eyes. "Do you have a little girl?" she asked.

"Yes, dear, I do," I answered. "And I never lie to her either."

Those big blue eyes melted my heart and brought me close to tears as she held her little arm up to me with the burned hand. "O.K.," she said.

My heart raced. "Please, God, let me get this line with one shot," I prayed. The needle slipped right in, and my brave patient never flinched. I made sure her blood pressure was high enough and then gave her morphine for the pain. She relaxed a little as I turned my attention to the sister. "I'm sorry I talked to you that way," I apologized. "Let's take care of you now." I pulled an emesis basin from the shelf and poured some sterile water into it to cool her feet. Her burns weren't serious, and she continued to help me care for her sister on the way to the hospital.

The baby was very groggy from the morphine by the time we arrived at the burn unit. On the way to the floor, she reached over, took my hand, and asked me if I was a hero like on TV. "No," I told her, "I'm just a mommy who goes to work in an ambulance."

I had always wondered what had happened to the two sisters. I don't check back on my patients very often; most of the time it's too painful. Nevertheless, here was their grandfather in the back of my ambulance, telling me the story. "How are the girls?" I asked.

"Oh fine," he said. "The little one has a few scars, but most of her hair grew back. The older one doesn't even have any scars." Looking back at me, he asked, "Do you know how I could get hold of that paramedic? I would sure like to thank her for what she did for my girls."

It was my turn to look out the window. "I'm sure she knows, sir." How could I tell him it was me? "I'm sure she knows and would be happy to hear the girls are O.K. Thank you for telling me about it."

By then we were at the hospital and took our patient up to his room. On the way back to quarters, my partner asked me if I was O.K. "You're awfully quiet," he said. "Did the old guy remind you of someone?"

"Yes," I told him. "The old guy reminded me of someone very special."

THANK YOU

I
t is not often that people in the field of emergency medicine hear *thank you*. They do not expect it because they are just doing the job they were intended to do. When someone does say thank you, it means so much. I remember the times when family and even patients expressed gratitude at the job I had done with humility and gratitude of my own.

People in crisis situations don't think about the rescuers and shouldn't. The rescuers have chosen the path they are on, and theirs is a life of emotional self-sacrifice. I once had a friend in the field who referred to it as a healthy expression of codependency. I agree for the most part, but it can be a self-destructive path also if those rampant emotions are not dealt with. People in emergency medicine have an inordinately large percentage of substance abuse, suicides, and disruptive family issues in their personal lives. There have arisen over the course of the years organizations to help these rescuers deal with some of the emotions they come across. Sometimes just talking to other rescuers helps relieve some of the pressure of what builds inside.

People who respond to the emergencies of others are usually honored to do so and consider the good they do to be enough. I did. But sometimes a simple acknowledgement of the fact that these people are there to help means more than all the paychecks or honors ever received.

"MOTHER'S DAY"

A friend had brought my kids to the station to visit. It was Mother's Day, and I had to work. It was one of the negatives of going into this line of work. Giving up the special days or celebrating them the next day. This was especially true since I was a single mom with bills to pay and no child support. Holidays paid overtime. I cuddled with my daughter on the couch and joked with my boys. They were the focus of my life and, since the divorce from their father, had been what kept me going no matter how tired I was. Mother's Day was special because of them, and I was so glad they could be with me—even if it meant time spent together at an ambulance station.

Our wonderful time ended with the loud pronouncement of tones ringing through the station. "Respond to a child versus motor vehicle." My heart sank. I kissed my babies good-bye as I ran to the rig.

We pulled up right behind the fire engine. The scene was chaos with hysterical people running in fifteen directions at once. I was still in paramedic school working as an EMT, and the medic I was working with yelled for me to set up the rig and explained that this was "load and go." I jumped in the back, pulled the monitor and an oxygen mask out, and got the IV's set up. In the few minutes it took the firefighter and my partner to wrap the unresponsive child on a board to protect her neck and back from further injury, I had the ambulance set and ready to go. I jumped out of the back as they climbed in. "Code three to County," my partner called. "Pediatric traumatic arrest."

My emotions were put on hold as I jumped in the front of the ambulance. Some well-meaning individual had placed the child's mother in the passenger seat. It was against company policy to transport anyone other than the patient when driving code three unless there were extenuating circumstances. It was just too risky. Her eyes met mine as I closed the door. It was Mother's Day. That was an extenuating circumstance in my heart.

I put the ambulance in gear and negotiated through the crowds of people in the street with the help of the police officers. The lights helped clear the way, and I played gently with the siren until we were clear of the crowd. Then it was full lights, sirens, and speed as I raced the hand of death toward the hospital.

The child's mother was unbelievably calm. I introduced myself and asked if she was O.K. "*Si,*" she responded. "Oh, I'm sorry. I mean yes; I am O.K." She told me her name was Maria and that her only daughter, who was obscured from our sight by three paramedics fighting to save her life, was two years old. "It wasn't her fault," she continued. "My sister, she is going to the store for more food. My baby, she is playing behind the car, and my sister did not see her. My family, we celebrate Mother's Day together." The story continued as I realized the horror of the moment. The family had all been together celebrating life and motherhood when one of the family members struck down this small child.

I glanced into the rearview mirror. My partner, Mike, was on the radio talking to the hospital, and I focused on his report while Maria continued with her story of celebrations and family. "County base, medic two. Two-year-old female, full arrest, severe head trauma with positive CSF both ears." My heart hurt to hear the words he spoke. I watched in the mirror as the paramedics did CPR on the tiny tot.

Maria reached out and patted my arm. "She will be O.K.," she said. "It is Mother's Day; a baby cannot die on Mother's Day."

I forced myself to focus on the driving as my mind recalled the lessons from paramedic school. A rate of 95 percent mortality for traumatic arrests. Severe head trauma. CSF, the abbreviation for cerebral spinal fluid. The baby had an open skull fracture. Her chances for survival were next to nothing. I looked again at Maria. She had a small smile on her face as she repeated the words that felt like stab wounds into my heart. "It is Mother's Day. She will not die today."

We had arrived at the hospital, and the medics in the back had unloaded the tiny patient and were already through the doors. I helped Maria get out of the ambulance and took her into the family waiting room. "Oh," she said, "this is nice. I thought I would have to wait in the lobby." I smiled at her. This is the room where they isolate the families who will hear bad news.

"I'll tell the nurses you're in here. They'll be with you soon." She didn't have to wait long. As I left the doorway, the doctor entered it with his head bowed and the burden of a mother's grief on his lips.

I went out to the ambulance and began cleaning the mess. Papers thrown everywhere. Blood. Too much blood for so tiny a child.

My partner walked out the back doors looking for the paperwork he would have to fill out. He looked in at me and spoke in anger. "You'd think those stupid people would learn to watch their kids."

I wanted to throw the bloody utensils at him. My eyes filled with tears even as I understood that the anger was his way of dealing with this tragedy. "Fuck you." I rarely cussed, and Mike did a double take.

"What? Oh God. I'm sorry," he said at the sight of my tears. Now I was angry. I threw open the side doors of the ambulance and climbed out. Slamming the doors behind me, I buried my head in my arms on the side of the ambulance. I fought the tears. I wanted to be angry. I did not want to feel the pain.

A hand touched my shoulder, and I swung angrily around. I was expecting Mike, and I wanted nothing more than to cut him to shreds with words. There was an EMT from another company standing there. Her name was Janet. That's all I knew about her.

"Do you smoke?" She said, offering me an already glowing cigarette.

"No," I stammered. I had quit a month ago. "Yes," I said as I reached out and took the cigarette. The smoke stung my healing lungs and eased the anger.

"I've got a shoulder too," she said. My mind fought against it, but my tears found her shoulder, and I cried. She understood.

"You know, why don't you go call your kids?" she said. "I'll clean up the rig for you."

I was never one to avoid my duty, but there was nothing I wanted more than to know that my children were home and safe by now—safe on Mother's Day. I found a pay phone around the corner and called the house. My son answered. I spoke very briefly to them, telling them I was checking to make sure they had arrived home O.K.

By the time I got back to the ambulance, Janet had cleaned and restocked the entire thing. "Thanks" was all I could muster.

She gave me a big hug. "Sometimes the guys don't understand," she said, handing me her home phone number. "Call me if you need to talk." With that she got in her own ambulance, and her partner drove off.

I had pulled it together by the time that Mike came back out. "You O.K.?" he asked rather sheepishly. I told him I was fine, and we headed back to quarters.

The next few hours were full of mind-numbing calls for which I was grateful. Stomachaches, headaches, a sprained ankle. I had started to relax when the radio spoke our number. "Emotional crisis" was the dispatch, and it was to the same address as the accident. Being sent code two meant that the police would beat us there. For that much I was relieved.

Our arrival was in the midst of the same crowd of relatives who had been at the horrible accident earlier in the day. We were directed to the kitchen of the house. One of the uniformed police officers was talking with a family member; the other seemed to be talking to a closet door.

"So what's going on?" my partner asked.

"There was an accident here earlier. A little girl was killed. The woman driving the car has locked herself in the closet and is refusing to come out." He ran his hand through his hair. "We may have to break down the door."

The officer speaking to the woman in the closet was threatening the same thing. "Listen, we can't leave you in there," he said. "Either you come out now or we break the door in."

I moved forward, my heart aching for this whole family, as Mike explained to the officers that we had transported the dying tot earlier. They did not need more violence here today.

"Officer, please let me try."

He looked me over brusquely, nodded his head in consent, and moved out of the way. "Her name is Theresa," he said.

Gently I tapped on the door. "Theresa? I'm with the ambulance. We need you to come out." Silence. I tried again and got the same response. The officers behind me were getting fidgety.

"Theresa? I understand. I want to help." Still silence. "Theresa? I'm a mother too."

As there was still no response, I started to move away to let the officers do things the way they knew. Slowly the door handle turned. Her pale, drawn face appeared in the back of the closet, the shroud of death that wasn't hers on her soul. The tear that had been fighting to escape all afternoon rolled slowly down my cheek at the sight of this woman's anguish. Theresa's eyes focused on the tear on my cheek, and her hand reached out to touch it. Her eyes found mine, and the question of understanding filled them. I opened my arms to her not saying a word, and Theresa's tears fell on my shoulder.

I learned an important lesson that day—one of the most important lessons of my paramedic training. Strength is replenished with the sharing of pain, and sometimes the only medication that will work is a shoulder to lean on.

"DUH"

It was late in the day, and we hadn't had a break yet. We had been running back-to-back calls all day long in the heat of summer. Tired and hungry, we had managed to grab a candy bar a few hours before at one of the hospitals but had been sent out—yet again—before relaxing with it. Half of my Snickers still sat uneaten on the dash shelf. My partner for the day was not a man used to missing meals. It showed. Dan was overweight and getting crankier by the minute as the day wore on. He had managed to grab a couple of bottles of water at the last hospital while I gave report, and I gratefully gulped one between bites of the remnants of my Snickers as we headed out.

Code two for a woman in labor, contractions ten minutes apart, second child. I glanced over at Dan, listening to him complain about the stupidity of the calls we had been on today. He was new, and I doubted he would be successful at making a career of this. It was not a job that allowed for comfortable living while on duty. Missed meals and no sleep for twenty-four hours made the best of us cranky at times. I was feeling it myself today. And he was right. The substance of the back-to-back calls today cumulatively did not equal an emergency. Still, this was what we had chosen to do for a living, and we did have days when we ate all we wanted and watched reruns of Andy Griffith and Opie all day long while lounging in air-conditioned quarters. Emergency medicine was completely unpredictable.

I swished the rest of the candy bar from my mouth as we pulled up to the scene. Neither of us was overly anxious to pull the gurney in this heat for contractions ten minutes apart. I grabbed the small bag that held my assessment tools, and we walked up to the door of an older ranch-style house on the frontage street. Chimes from the doorbell were answered by a man's taunting voice from within the house. "Sandy, your ride is here."

And the answering female voice: "God damn it, Ray, I'm feeding the kid. You get it."

The man's voice responded, "I ain't your fuckin' slave. Get it yourself."

And the woman's voice: "They can just wait then."

What little patience I had was holding on by a thread as I watched Dan's face go red. He started pounding on the door with his fist. "We can hear you out here, and we are not just going to wait," he yelled. "You want a ride to the hospital? Open the door now, or we are leaving and sending the cops instead."

Movement through the side window of the door showed the owner of the male voice as he moved off the couch, remote in one hand and beer in the other. The door was thrown open, and he—without diverting his eyes from the TV—jabbed toward the open kitchen. "She's in there," he said.

The house was hot even with the doors open, and the smell of stale food and bad socks permeated the air. Sitting at the Formica kitchen table was an obviously pregnant woman feeding a squirming and unhappy two year old bites of macaroni and cheese.

Stepping around a pile of dirty clothes in the doorway, I addressed the woman. "Ma'am, you called for an ambulance?"

"Come on, Junior, one more bite for Mommy." She plunged the spoon of macaroni in the unhappy face.

"Excuse me, ma'am," I tried again. "We are with the ambulance, and someone called the emergency line to request us for a woman in labor. Would that be you?"

Not looking up at me, she proceeded to scoop yet another spoonful of mac and cheese into the resisting Junior's mouth. "Course it's me. Do you see any other pregnant woman around here?" she queried. "Junior, eat!"

The now bright-red Dan stepped around me, and I let him. "Look, lady. You called; we came. Now we go with or without you," he huffed.

Finally we had her attention. "Well, you are a rude one!" The tray with Junior's mac and cheese was forgotten. Junior started wailing as Mommy yelled at Dan. This day was just getting longer and longer.

"Ma'am," I said, putting a restraining hand on Dan's arm. "Do you want an ambulance or not? The town is very busy today."

Looking me up and down, Junior's mom scooped the rest of the food into the already full sink. "I guess I called you, didn't I?" She waddled over to the doorway of the living room and addressed the man on the couch. "Ray! Get your ass up and get my bag." Ray just grunted as she waddled back over and scooped Junior from his chair. With no pause, she redirected to us. "And I know the law, so don't give me any guff. You have to take me to the hospital because I called you." Grabbing a filthy dishcloth, she scrubbed the screaming child with it. "We have to go by the store first and get some formula, and then we can drop off Junior at Mom's on the way."

Dan stood staring with his checks puffed and his ears and neck the color of boiled lobster. I quickly grabbed his arm and pulled him back next to me. "Dan, go set up the gurney for me will you, please?" I said, moving around in front of him. As Dan quickly made a steamy retreat, I approached the mother of screaming Junior. "Ma'am, this is an emergency vehicle. We don't run errands." I tried holding my hands out in a manner of supplication.

She turned her angry eyes to mine. "Listen, you, I know the law, and you are taking me, or I'll have your job." Taking a deep breath, I blamed her hormones so I could stay rational and tried again. "Listen, ma'am. We don't do errands. This vehicle is dedicated to running *emergencies!* Yes, we will take you to the hospital, but we will not help you with your shopping or haul Junior to the sitters. *That* would cost us our jobs. If you would like to argue that fact, we can have a police officer come explain it to you while we actually run some emergency calls." I stood my ground calmly as she pushed her pregnant belly into me. We were about the same height, and we stood eye to eye for a while.

"Oh, fine!" she huffed, breaking away. "Ray, go get Elaine from next door," she said, pushing around me and shuffling through the pile of laundry.

Ray had put down his beer and stood by the front door watching the ambulance sway as Dan readied the back. He headed out the door as Junior's mom tossed the toddler unceremoniously into the playpen that sat in the corner of the living room. She disappeared down the hallway and came back in just a few minutes lugging a baby bag stuffed to overflowing. Shoving the bag and her medical card at me, she aimed her bulk across the lawn toward Ray and Elaine.

All three came shuffling across the lawn, and I headed out to the rig for a few deep breaths before we began this ride. I had hoped she would be going to one of the closer facilities, but the card she handed me as I walked out the door indicated the county hospital. From where we were, that meant ten minutes through town and then a twenty-minute ride down the freeway to the other side of town. I stuck my head in the front and told Dan we were headed for County, and then I went around to the back and waited.

It seemed that Ray was coming along for the ride, a practice that was discouraged for safety reasons, but I was already past my patience limit and figured it would be easier to haul him along than to try to reason with the pregnant one. I walked back to the front and opened the door for Ray, avoiding the caustic looks that Dan was shooting my way. My huge patient had crawled into the back of the ambulance and was trying to maneuver her giant bulk around by the time I got her hubby tucked into the front. I climbed in the back after her.

"Your medical card identifies you as Sandy. Is that the name you go by?" I asked, trying to soften the tension in my voice.

"Yes." Without acknowledging my presence with so much as a glance, Sandy adjusted herself in the seat. As I reached out to take her arm for a blood pressure, she jerked away from me. "What do you think you are doing?" she demanded.

"Well, Sandy, this is an ambulance, and I am a paramedic." Sarcasm oozed out before I could stop it. "I am now going to take your blood pressure and pulse rate, and then you are going to answer my questions so that I can tell the hospital what is going on. That is the way this works."

Sandy stared hard at me. "I only want a ride," she said.

She had reached my limit, and you could hear it in my voice. "One more time: that is not the way this works."

Acquiescence was not a natural talent of Sandy's. She huffed her cheeks, stared out the back, and answered my questions with single words.

"When are you due, Sandy?"

"July."

"Sandy, it's June."

She looked right at me. "Duh."

Glancing out the front, I was glad to see we were pulling onto the freeway. Twenty minutes to go. "Are you sure you're in labor?"

Again, she stared me down. "Duh."

I was really starting to feel sorry for Ray in the front. "Sandy, when was your last contraction?"

Sandy again looked me straight in the eye, only instead of a repeat of her eloquent answers, her face slowly pulled back in a frightening grimace. "*Yyyyeeeeeaaaaaaaaawwww*!!" Sandy screamed. The ambulance jerked as Dan reacted. Glancing down at Sandy's legs, I watched her sweatpants start to bulge between her now widespread legs.

"Crap. Dan, get over to the side. I need your help now," I yelled, reaching up for the OB kit over Sandy's head. The ambulance rocked hard as Dan pulled to the side of the busy freeway and slammed on the brakes.

Ray's horrified face appeared momentarily through the gap between the front and the back of the ambulance. "Sandy!" he screamed, and then I heard two doors slam.

Reaching down, I grabbed Sandy's sweatpants, and as she screamed again, pulled hard. There between her legs was the baby. I glanced up as Dan swung open the back doors of the ambulance. Sandy was now exposed to the world. "Dan, close the doors!" I yelled, but Dan was distracted as Ray brushed by him and ran past the back of the ambulance. "Catch that guy before he gets killed!"

Grabbing the sides of the OB kit, I ripped it open and removed the bulb that I used to suction the baby's nose and mouth. I looked up again to see Ray run past the gap in the rear doors of the ambulance with Dan in hot pursuit. They were literally running circles around the ambulance on the side of the freeway. "Dan!" I yelled as I reached for the umbilical clamps, Sandy still screaming in the background. Ray again whizzed by the back doors, and five steps behind, my red-faced, out-of-shape partner huffed in hot pursuit.

Sandy's screaming cut off abruptly as the liver-colored placenta plopped out onto the gurney beside the squirming, now screaming baby. Again, Ray ran by, and now at least half an ambulance behind, my partner followed in hot pursuit, bright red with sweat flying off of him. I quickly clipped and cut the umbilicus, wrapping the baby in the paper blankets provided in the delivery kit. Sandy had stopped yelling and was staring out the back door at the circular foot race of her husband and my partner as they sweated and grunted past again. Dan was losing ground, and I figured Ray would be passing him soon.

Handing the newborn infant to his now quiet mother and covering her with a blanket to keep the interstate from seeing things best not seen on the daily commute, I ripped off my bloodied gloves and jumped out the back door. *Wham!* Dan hit me hard, and if I hadn't been holding onto the door, I might have fallen. Then two seconds later Ray bounced off Dan's back, effectively halting his purposeless race and landing him on his keister in the gravel on the side of the road.

Dan was bent over at the rear door of the ambulance, dripping wet and struggling to breathe as Ray sat stunned on the side of the road. Sandy, now cuddling her newborn infant, started to laugh. Great whoops of laughter. I walked over to Ray and helped him to his feet. Brushing the debris off his bottom, I helped him into the jump seat in the back of the ambulance behind his hysterically giggling wife and their new baby.

Dan waved a hand at us, slammed the back doors, and stumbled back to the front of the ambulance to continue the journey to County.

"O.K., Sandy, what didn't you tell me?" I asked as I removed the blanket and scooped up the still-warm placenta to place it in a plastic bag for later examination.

Still giggling and now nursing her newborn, Sandy said, "The doctors cut out three quarters of my cervix after Junior was born. I guess that matters, huh?"

Now it was my turn to say it. "Duh."

EIGHTY YEARS

He had started dating her when he was eighteen years old and she was sixteen. He told me it was love at first sight and that the secret to their longevity was never going to bed mad. His eyes glowed when he looked at her in a way that I will never forget and still envy.

I had responded on a transfer to another hospital. He was going to Sacramento for heart surgery. They wouldn't do it at the hospital he was at because of his age. He was a large man with broad shoulders and a smile that made me forget the negativity I had brought to work with me.

I had just ended a relationship with a man who harbored so much anger that I could still feel the resonance of it in my soul some days.

My patient introduced himself to me as Ed and asked me if it would be possible for his wife to ride along with us. Although my mind screamed that I did not want the intrusion today, his smile found me blaming the policies of the company I worked for and making obligatory excuses.

"Oh, that's O.K.," he sighed. "I only asked because it is our anniversary and my little lady had made plans that I messed up with this silly heart thing. I'm sure she will understand." He reached over and patted the wrinkled hand that rested on the chrome rail of the bed that held him. Tears glistened in the eyes that smiled toward the man in the bed as his wife nodded her consent. "Yes, my love, there is always next year."

Their smiles and obvious love loosened the bars that were wrapped around my heart by my latest misadventure at romance.

"Well, I guess it would be O.K. if she rode in the front." My partner stared at me open-eyed in disbelief.

My patient's wife stood by the bedside but could have been a patient herself. Her back was rounded with the years, and her hair gathered into a bun that rested upon those shoulders. She leaned on a cane, obviously fatigued from spending so many hours in the emergency room, and a slight quiver shook her.

Maneuvering himself into a position where he could ask me without anyone else hearing, my anguished partner whispered, "Just how am I supposed to get Grandma into the rig?" The ambulance was built on a Ford 350 chassis and rode high.

I felt tired and just wanted to get this transfer over. "I don't know. Use the code steps," I said, pointing to the small step stool in the room that allowed for elevation when chest compressions were performed.

I removed the hospital's wires and equipment from my patient and hooked the portable equipment to him as the RN gave me a report on his impending surgery. "Thanks for taking the wife. They're a special couple."

My depressive fatigue just didn't care as I took the paperwork and we loaded the gurney into the rear of the ambulance. My partner used the code step and two nurses to get the fragile wife into the front seat, shooting me daggers with his eyes at the added trouble. Radio numbers were given, and the ambulance began the rocking journey to another city.

"You O.K., snookums?" The little gray head tried to peek around the bulkhead that separated the old lady from her love.

"Doin' fine, sweetums. Don't you worry your little head."

Exhaustion and disillusionment clouded my soul, but I had to ask, "How long have you two been together?"

"Today is our eightieth wedding anniversary, but I've been in love with that woman since the day I laid eyes on her. Her daddy wanted to kill me when I told him I was going to marry that girl. Had to run off to be together, but we made it. I got the girl, and she has always been my strength."

What an incredible strength it spoke of. Headed for heart surgery at ninety-eight years old with the woman of his dreams on their eightieth wedding anniversary. I was amazed and enraptured as he proceeded to tell me tales of their early years out east and their move to California, "the land of opportunity." I chuckled as he used the tired cliché. He spoke of not having enough and of having plenty after he started working for the railroad. He spoke of their children with pride and their achievements with the passion that made them his own. Always his story curved around and sped back to touch the rock that was his life, the silver-haired woman in the front with my partner.

For over an hour I listened, captured by tales of his life and undying love for his soul's partner, who had made the journey with him. He still seemed in awe of the love that he had found as a child and followed through life.

We arrived safely at our destination and waited while my partner convinced two EMTs from another company to help get "sweetums" out of the ambulance safely and up the ramp to the doors. Ed and his love held hands as we made our way through the halls of the hospital and to the cardiac ward at a pace that caused my partner's face to darken and his shoulders to hunch. Transferring their care, as it had always been the two of them, I bade them luck and explained the special day to the nurse caring for them.

"What were you thinking?" My partner didn't wait to get back to the rig before he voiced his concerns of liability and safety. I knew he couldn't understand because he had not seen the look on Ed's face when he spoke of his Emma. I didn't understand fully, but I sure hoped that someday I would.

"Just give me this one, O.K.?" I pulled the door closed behind me and turned my head so my partner couldn't intrude on the remnants of Ed's story, which coursed through my heart.

LOVE

One of the most compelling aspects of working in emergency medicine is the ongoing confrontation with raw emotion. Fear, anger, and denial, but also trust, love, and faith are all exposed in their raw forms. To witness life at its peaks and valleys can be as rewarding as it is frightening.

I have always been profoundly affected by the couples that survive life together. Through it all they manage the hills and valleys and stay as one. I began years ago to ask the secret to success, questioning only as someone who finds the mystery beyond her grasp. The answers varied. Mostly I was told to value friendship and forget anger before bedtime. Once in a while I met a couple who, when they looked at each other, glowed as if electrified. They didn't seem to know the answer. They just were. The number of years shared didn't seem to matter. There was a connection, a life force that existed.

I have been in love. Most of us have. We have all dreamed of someone to spend a lifetime with, no matter what the Fates throw at us. Few of us have achieved it. I have been witness to some relationships that made it look easy. My fleeting glimpse of a love that sustains has been enough to make hope spring eternal in my heart that someday I will meet the one that is my constant.

Love is one of the most powerful motivators for life, hope, and drama. I have seen it unfold in tragic consequences that befuddled the mind with anger and death, tearing people from the pages of life because of their need to be with someone who would not or could not love them back. I have seen the jealousy that consumes reality and causes the walls of decency to crumble, the rawest forms of betrayal, and the heartbreak that is left behind. And I have stolen an occasional glimpse at the fluid magic that has inspired poetry through the ages with the strength of commitment that I could only envy.

Addendum: I eventually did find this amazing form of love in my life. It was at a time when I had stopped looking. He is my husband and the love of my life. He is also my muse, and it is to him and my children that this book is dedicated.

THE GUY IN THE CORNER

It was Friday at noon. It had been a busy day so far, though none of the calls had been extraordinary. My partner, Troy, and I were sitting in quarters, eating lunch and hoping for an hour or so of downtime. Of course, wishing for downtime pretty much guaranteed it wasn't going to happen. I hadn't even finished my sandwich when the lights blinked on and the tones sounded. "Medic twelve, engine fifteen, respond code three to Marrows Restaurant at Magnolia and the interstate for an altered level and difficulty breathing."

I've learned to dread these types of calls in restaurants, especially at lunchtime. Even a simple call can get complicated when there are crowds of people around. Hopefully this would be something easy. The location was only a block or so from the fire station of engine fifteen, and we were several miles away through downtown traffic. Engine fifteen was manned with at least one medic. I was hopeful that they would have the patient stabilized and ready to go by the time we got there. We could transport and still get back to quarters in time for a short rest before the evening rush of calls.

It took us about four minutes to get within sight of the restaurant. The parking lot was packed with cars. I hoped my intuition was wrong and the patient would not be too seriously ill. We had to pull slightly past Marrows and then make a U-turn to get into the parking lot. Just as we made the turn to enter the parking lot, the captain on engine fifteen came up on the radio. "Cancel medic twelve and send us the coroner."

This was not right! Calling for the coroner meant that there was nothing that could be done for this patient. That just didn't make sense. The inside of the restaurant was obviously packed with people. How could anyone have died and remained unnoticed long enough for the paramedics on the engine to be unable to do anything for him?

Troy looked over at me as he shut off the lights and siren. "Make any sense to you?" he asked. "That place is packed."

"No," I answered, "but there are medics on that engine. They wouldn't have called it unless there was nothing to be done." We had already made the U-turn for the driveway. "Troy, let's at least stop and take them a sheet," I said. "They don't have anything with them to cover the body with. We can at least provide them with some privacy while they wait."

Troy turned the ambulance into the driveway of the restaurant and parked it behind the engine. It usually took a while for a coroner's van to show up, and most people have never seen a dead body. People don't react very well to the sight, especially in a public place. Unlike in the movies, human beings are not a pretty sight when they have died.

I walked around to the back of the ambulance and pulled out one of our extra sheets. I handed it to Troy, and we walked toward the door. I had just opened the first door to the entrance when the captain of the engine met us in the opening. "I canceled you guys. The wife produced DNR papers."

It still didn't make much sense. A DNR is a set of papers that states a patient's wishes should something happen to him or her. It usually means that the person was expecting to die soon and did not wish any heroic measures be taken to prolong his or her life—an understandable measure. When the heart stops, the measures taken to get it going again can be very traumatic and are not always 100 percent successful. However, death takes a while to happen, even in someone who is terminally ill. The body doesn't usually die all at once. The drive to survive is powerful, with the body attempting to take breaths even after the heart has stopped.

"We brought you a sheet," I explained. "This place looks crowded, and we thought you might want to cover him up until the coroner gets here."

"We don't need it," the captain responded. "We have the guy propped up in a chair against the wall."

I glanced at my partner. This still didn't make sense. Dead people look dead. Why traumatize the whole restaurant—not to mention the man's wife? Why turn the man into a spectacle? Even if he had died, the body should be treated with respect. Troy offered the captain the sheet again. "We thought you might want to cover him up," Troy said, trying again.

"We don't need it." The captain glanced around. "We have him sitting in a chair, propped up against the wall. No one will notice."

I wanted to say, "You have got to be kidding me," but obviously he wasn't. Dead people look dead. Of course people will notice. I tried again. "Captain, do you want to put him on the gurney and move him to the ambulance until the coroner's van gets here?" The captain looked back into the crowded restaurant. "No," he said, "the coroner will be here soon. He's sitting right behind this wall in a chair. We've got him propped up. We don't want to tie you guys up."

Troy and I turned and walked back to the ambulance. We were both in disbelief. Human beings are funny creatures, but to prop a dead or dying man against a wall in a restaurant and think no one would notice was a new one for both of us.

We were silent as we turned back onto the road and headed back to our quarters. Both of us were a little shocked. "I can't believe that just happened," I said. "I thought I had seen everything."

Troy was silent for a while more. "Disgusting jokes now or later?" he asked. Humor was a strong survival mechanism in emergency medicine. It kept workers from hurting too bad when things didn't make sense.

"Now," I said. "I need to be distracted."

Troy grinned slowly. "I bet the restaurant gets stiffed with the bill."

I snickered. This was going to get bad. "You know," I said, "I hear their coffee is to die for."

Troy chuckled. "They've also got a killer salad bar," he responded.

I laughed. My turn: "Excuse me, waitress. I'll have whatever the guy in the corner *did not* have."

Troy: "I bet the waitress gets really angry when she asks him if he wants more coffee and he won't answer." Then in a squeaky high voice: "He's not only quiet and rude, but I'll bet he leaves a lousy tip!"

Me: "Excuse me, miss. Could we have *a lot* of ice for the guy in the corner?"

"You know, miss, most restaurants just have potted plants in the corner."

By now we were both holding our stomachs with laughter. It helped. We still didn't believe what had just happened, but the laughter helped.

BURNOUT

There is a phenomenon in medical care that is called burnout. I have known people who felt they had it, and I have known people considered burned out. I have even felt a little burned out myself at times (although it was usually nothing that a weekend at the beach or in the mountains wouldn't cure).

A wise woman who owned and operated a professional ambulance service for thirty years once told me that burnout is just an excuse. After twenty years in this business, I have to agree with her. I think it is an excuse. On the positive side, it is an excuse to take some time off and relax with friends and family. Unfortunately, it is also an excuse to be lazy and mean to people.

There is nothing more aggravating than to see a medical provider treat a patient poorly, although I am sure that I have not always been the picture of understanding and comfort. At three o'clock in the morning on your third call for a sore throat or a sprained ankle, it is hard to be wonderfully comforting. The problem with fatigue—burnout—is that you turn off that little voice that tells you the truth about what the patient is telling you. As anyone who works with the public will tell you, at times the communication that speaks the loudest is nonverbal. Allowing yourself to become tired, fatigued, or burned out runs the risk of not recognizing the underlying rhythm of what is really being said.

Those who serve the public in need all share the same symptoms of this type of behavior. I think we become so used to the pace of what we do and the expected interaction with our patients that we begin to see through a hazy fog. Are all the homeless people who say they have chest pain just looking for a free meal? And are the chronic-care patients drug seekers just because they know the dose and drug that gives them relief? Are we going to fix their addiction by denying them one dose of a medication?

A key to happiness in life is to determine a solution at the same time we recognize a problem. I do not know the solution to burnout. People are not emotionally designed for a job that involves sadness and pain every day. The heart needs balance—laughter to balance the tears and joy to balance anger.

There are wiser people than I who have tried to create a system that could differentiate between the man who gets a prescription for Vicodin so he can sell it on the street corner for five dollars a pill and the man who lies awake in pain because the doctor didn't give him an extra six pills to get him through the night. Perhaps the man didn't present as if he was really in pain, having lived with it for years. His blood pressure has learned to compensate, as has his heart rate.

To see the extent of human suffering every day and wish in your heart to fix it all can tarnish even the most sterling of characters after a few years. Nevertheless, the homeless person with the chest pain may be focused on a sandwich and not his heart attack because he hasn't had anything clean to eat in two days.

THE BATTLE OF THE BOOBS

Her name was Lacretia, and she had earned the reputation as a "frequent flyer."

It was a term for people who abused the welfare system by calling ambulances for rides to the hospital for nonemergency situations. These people had learned through the years that the Medi-Cal system in California was not policed with the same efficiency as most insurance programs, and therefore it was cheaper to call an ambulance for a ride than to call a taxi. There was also the mistaken belief that taking an ambulance to the hospital guaranteed you a bed in the ER no matter how busy the hospital was. It may have been so at one point in history, but because of the abuse the system suffered, even ambulance patients were triaged, and the nonemergency ones were sent to the lobby to wait their turn like everyone else.

Lacretia was a relatively healthy individual who lived off the welfare system. The closest we had come to witnessing an emergency with Lacretia was the last time we had seen her. That day she had been in an argument with her boyfriend, and he had thrown an egg at her. When we had arrived, she was waiting on the porch with her Medi-Cal card in hand demanding a ride to the hospital. She had refused an examination and become so abusive that we had to call for PD backup. Once the police officers were on scene, she told us she had an eggshell in her eye but still refused to allow us to look. It had escalated to the point where the officers had threatened to arrest her when she finally allowed us to look at her eye. It was an incredible sight. The entire back half of the eggshell had somehow inverted and sealed itself to her left eye like a giant white contact lense. We took her to the hospital with both eyes bandaged and two police officers in tow.

Today we had been sent code two for an unknown problem. Lacretia was notorious for calling 911 and demanding an ambulance without giving a reason. We knew her address by heart and neither my partner nor I was looking forward to another encounter.

We pulled up in front of Lacretia's brand new home. Part of the city's urban redevelopment plan, it was quite impressive from the front even though the lawn that had been planted with such high hopes was already dying from neglect and suffocation under piles of garbage. Erin, my partner, grabbed the trauma bag and stomped up to the front door.

Erin was a tall man in his forties who had made a career out of EMS. He had a great sense of humor, but it rarely showed on the job. Instead he projected a dignified, stoic type of personality. He was a great medic but had little tolerance for people who abused the system. Lacretia was one of his least favorites. She answered the door on the first knock. She was packed and ready to go, Medi-Cal card in one hand and a huge bag packed with snacks and trashy romance novels in the other. Lacretia was a large woman, but she loved her spandex. Tonight she wore black leotards that pulled at the seams and a stretched-tight tube top while trying to maintain some semblance of dignity. The top was one of simple strapless design that wrapped around her upper chest and was held in place by her breasts. Lacretia was well endowed in that area, and the tube top pulled as tightly as the pants.

My partner spoke to her with weariness. "Lacretia, what's the problem today?"

She responded by snorting through her nose. "I's got a spida bite," she replied as she pulled the door shut behind her. "Lez go."

Erin shook his head as he watched her. "Lacretia, we went through this last time. We have to know what is going on so that we can call the hospital on the radio and tell them what's wrong with you." Erin's patience was thin tonight, and you could hear it in his voice as he spoke to her. "We need to know what kind of spider it was, Lacretia."

Lacretia turned on her heels, pushed her face directly into Erin's and shouted, "How the hell am I supposed to know what kin' o' spida it was? One wit eight legs I guess. I never saw it."

Erin placed his hand on her shoulder to maintain the distance. "Lacretia, we don't want to argue with you again. Remember how bad it got last time with the police. Now I need you to tell me about the bite."

Lacretia pulled back and looked Erin up and down. "I remembers you. You's a smart ass that called the po-po on me. Well, I's gots a spida bite, and you's takin' me to the hospital. I knows da rules. You's got to take me. I never seen no spida, but I woke up and I's got a bite on me, and I's goin' to the hospital in da amblance."

Erin's patience was gone, but he maintained the calm voice and demeanor. "Lacretia, I need to see the spider bite."

She dropped her bags where she stood. "I could die here waitin' for you. I's got a spida bite, and now you wants to see it. O.K. It's right here." With that statement, Lacretia grabbed the bottom of her tube top and yanked it up to her shoulders. Like two live amoebas free from their confines, her huge breasts bounced up and down with the exertion, fully exposed to the world and threatening to strike my partner in the face if she moved any closer. They seemed to have obtained a life of their own. The miracle of the spandex age came to reality as the freed entities swung and danced before Erin's eyes. I tried not to stare as the phrase "two cats in a gunny sack" played in my head—only these two were loose and still fighting. And these were more in the bobcat size range.

Erin's dignified stance was gone. His jaw dropped open, and his eyes were as large as pie plates. The color drained from his face. He turned and walked down the steps, dropping the trauma bag. Like a man blinded by a light that's too bright, he walked past without see-ing me. "You had better take this one," he mumbled.

I stepped up on the landing with Lacretia and with some diffi-culty pulled her top back in place.

"Wa's the matter wit him? He never seen a boob before? I done got's a spida bite right here," she said, yanking the tube top back up and freeing her breasts from their cage. The wild animals were again unleashed as she pointed to a small red mark about three inches above her left nipple.

"O.K., Lacretia," I said as I once again reached out and adjusted the stressed fabric back down over her still bouncing breasts. "Why don't we go get in the ambulance and head for the hospital?"

I turned and walked to the ambulance with Lacretia on my heels. "Don' you wants to see my spida bite?"

I was afraid to acknowledge her question as I opened the back doors and climbed in, adjusting the gurney for the ride. Lacretia climbed in behind me and plopped herself on the bed. She reached down and fastened the seat belt herself as Erin closed the back doors without looking up and headed for the hospital.

The trip was a nightmare of fighting spandex and bouncing breasts as Lacretia insisted on showing me her "spida bite" three or four times. I battled to keep the spandex down long enough to obtain a blood pressure and pulse rate. There was no inflammation of the site where she claimed the spider had "attacked" her, and I managed to get the information that she had seen a "big spida" in her living room the previous night and then woke up with the small red mark on her breast. Explaining to her that the bite didn't appear serious at the time reassured her to the point that the spandex stayed in place, and the battle of the bounce was restrained by the time we arrived at the ER.

Lacretia undid her seat belt and was waiting when Erin opened the back doors. He never looked at her as he turned and led her into the hospital corridor. Opening the door to the triage area, he quickly told her to sign in and closed the self-locking door before she could turn back. Lacretia pounded on the door. "Wa's you doin'?" she screamed on the other side of the door. "I's got a spida bite. I done come by amblance, and I don' have to go out here!"

The lobby of the ER was packed, and Lacretia, in no immediate danger, had been sent to wait for an available bed along with the people who had driven themselves to the hospital. I was explaining the situation to the triage nurse when a clerk came running into the room. "Where's security?" she asked. "There's a woman going nuts out there." She looked horrified as she ran down the corridor in search of the security officer. Erin and I looked at each other and then went into the registration area that was surrounded by bulletproof glass.

There in the lobby stood Lacretia. This time the restrictive spandex was pulled completely off, and the freedom of the fighting breasts was assured as she danced around in the lobby. Illnesses and injuries were temporarily forgotten by the waiting numbers at the sight of Lacretia's breasts as she angrily addressed anyone within listening distance. Even through the glass we could hear her screaming. "I's gots a spida bite! I's gots a spida bite!" The normal hum of conversation had died away completely, reminding me of the quiet in a forest when a predator is on the prowl. Lacretia's breasts were the only things moving in the lobby, and her screams were the only sound.

Security had arrived and frozen in the doorway at the imminent battle before them. To restrain the woman was one thing, but those breasts seemed to have a life of their own. The two officers stood mute with the same look on their faces as Erin's at his first introduction to the beasts.

The triage nurse rushed from her room, freeing the security officers from their trance. Lacretia was not to be reasoned with and was finally led into a small waiting area in the back of the ER to await her turn. I only wish I had been there when the unsuspecting emergency-room doctor asked her, "What's wrong with you tonight?"

"MY COUNTRY 'TIS OF THEE"

W orking the downtown area again. They had termed it the "knife-and-gun club"; it had a history of being violent. This town was the farthest inland port on the California coast and dated back to the days of the gold rush. It had always been a rough-and-tumble kind of a town. This was the lowest rent district, and most of the shelters for the homeless were down here.

It was the weekend before the Fourth of July during a very hot summer, and the call volume had been typical for the area. Homeless people didn't do well in the 110-degree heat. We had spent most of the day taking dehydrated homeless alcoholics out to County Hospital. This call didn't appear to be any different from the rest. PD on scene, ETOH ground-level fall. That was the radio lingo for drunks who had fallen down either from their level of inebriation, dehydration, or other causes to be determined by the medics and the doctors we took them to.

The location was easy enough to find. Just a few blocks down from our station, it was on the main street that stretched the width of the city between two interstates. There were two police cars parked next to the curb with their lights flashing to mark the location. One of the officers leaned up against his car, watching his comrades deal with the man I assumed was destined to be our patient.

He was around fifty, and the years of alcohol abuse and life on the streets showed in the lines in his face. The fatigue jacket he wore maintained its stubborn army green under the layers of street dirt it carried, and the fresh darkening on its collar bore witness to the blood that oozed from a matted area in the man's greasy hair. It had been worn brown around the bottom, and the front pocket on the left was ripped, showing its black liner. Our new patient was obviously not a happy drunk, gesturing and yelling at the police officers. He was in the process of guessing the species of one of the officer's mothers as we walked up.

"Evening, officers." My partner addressed the guardians of our patient. "What can we do for you?"

The officer leaning on the car answered the question. "Joe took a tumble. He's got a nasty gash on his head tonight. We need you guys to take him to County for an eval before we let him sleep it off."

"No problem." My partner, a tall, burly-looking guy with an easy attitude, walked up to the group gathered on the sidewalk next to an empty alley.

"Joe, they tell me you fell. Let's have a look—"

"Fuck you," said Joe as he swung at my partner. "You communist."

Joe had obviously been celebrating the Fourth of July in advance. He was too drunk to stand up without weaving, let alone fight anyone, and the exertion from the swing nearly sent him into the side of the building.

One of the officers started to move in on Joe. "Come on, Joe. We can do this the hard way or the easy way."

Joe's head rolled back on his neck, showing a crease of black as he tried to focus on the officer. "I have always done things the hard way. You want to make something of it?"

As the officer reached for his handcuffs, I decided that maybe I should intervene. Sometimes aggressive men reacted better to female paramedics.

"Officer, let me try," I said. I then addressed Joe, trying to use my most nonconfrontational voice. "Joe, you've got a cut on your head. We need to look at it."

Joe rolled his head back around and viewed me up and down. "So now the woman gets involved. Fuck you too, you communist."

Feigning insult, I placed my hands on my hips. "How dare you! Do you think you're a better American then I am, Joe?"

"Did you fight in the war?" Joe yelled. "Did you watch your friends die?"

I yelled right back at Joe as the officers hid their amusement. "No, Joe, I didn't. But I pick up veterans every day I work, and I can tell you right now I have more respect for you than you do."

Joe's head rolled again as he eyed me up and down. "Oh, she thinks she's tough.," he said, crossing his arms in front of his chest. "You want me to go to the hospital? You try and make me."

Holding my hand up to quiet one of the officers who was getting antsy, I walked over to Joe and put my arm around his shoulders. The odor of day-old booze and days or weeks of human sweat on an unwashed body was horrific, and I tried to breathe from the side of my mouth and away from Joe as I spoke. "Joe, between you and me, I don't have to make you do anything. I'm here to give you a ride to the hospital in a nice clean ambulance. You want to go with me or with the officers?" Joe's reaction was to swing at my face with his free hand. The alcohol slowed Joe's reflexes horribly, and it was an easy blow to avoid. I ducked and came up dancing in my best imitation of the great Ali, punching the air around me in a mock shadow box. "You think you're tough, Joe? Come on, come on—" I said as I danced, the officers and my partner looking on with a mix of shock and complete disbelief. "Come on, Joe," I continued, borrowing lines from my son's favorite musical. "Come on. I'll fight ya with one hand tied behind my back...I'll fight ya with my eyes closed."

Joe's eyes had widened at my performance, and now his aged face cracked with a smile. He winked his eyes at me as he pulled his head back. "Hey, I like you. You're all right." He said, punching me in the shoulder gently. Then he addressed the officers who were now laughing in a restrained officer fashion. "O.K., I'll go with them but only if the crazy woman is in the back with me." The officers laughed even harder as my partner and I put Joe on the gurney, and I climbed into the back with him.

My partner started the well-worn trip to County Hospital as I quickly took Joe's blood pressure and pulse rate. Suddenly Joe pushed me away again. "Hey, are you a communist?" he said, squinting his eyes at me.

"No, Joe, I'm not a communist," I said as I wrote down his vital signs on the paperwork.

"You're a fucking communist!" Joe yelled, reaching for the seatbelt release. My hands shot out to stop him from releasing the catch, and Joe caught me in the side of the head with his free hand. "You're a goddamned communist!" he yelled as we wrestled.

"Wrong!" I yelled at Joe. "You're the communist. You just hit a woman! Only communists hit women."

My partner had started to pull the ambulance to the side of the road to get into the back and help. I waved him to continue as Joe pulled back in shocked disbelief that I had called him a communist.

"I am not a Communist!" he said, obviously horrified that I would think such a thing. "I'm an American."

"Good Americans don't hit women," I countered.

Joe rolled his head back again and looked at me along the bridge of his nose, fighting for focus. He stared at me for a minute in disbelief then crossed his arms angrily. "You don't know nothing about bein' an American," he muttered. Suddenly Joe began singing at the top of his lungs, his drunken voice echoing around the rear of the, *"Oh, say can you see..."*

My partner glanced nervously in the rear view mirror assuring my safety.

"by the dawns early light..."

Joe was reaching for the straps again to undo them. *"What so proudly we hailed..."*

I reached out, took Joe's hands in mine, and joined him in his stanza *"at the twilight's last gleaming"* Joe starred at me again as we continued our chorus. His drunken bass voice and my Alto, *"Whose broad strips and bright stars through the perilous fight..."*

My partner's eyes met mine in the rear view mirror and he shook his head and smiled. Whatever it takes. *"O'r the ramparts we watched were so gallantly streaming."*

Joe voice became louder still and his arms reached out to direct the band playing in his head as we neared our crescendo, *"And the rockets' red glare, the bombs bursting in air, gave proof through the night that our flag was still there."*

Joe dropped my hand and with tears now streaming down his soiled face flailed his arms about, directing with all his energy. *"OH, SAY DOES THAT STAR-SPANGLED BANNER YET WAVE, O'ER THE LAND OF FREE—AND THE HOME OF THE BRAVE."*

Joe's hands dropped to his lap as he bowed his head. His eyes remained closed with the tears streaming down his face.

We had arrived at the county hospital, and as my partner opened the rear doors, Joe lifted his head. Looking at my partner through his alcohol-glazed eyes, he muttered, "Communist." Then Joe turned and looked at me. "I like you. You're a good person."

"You are too, Joe. You need to treat yourself like it."

Joe smiled and shook his life-weary head. "Seen too much," he muttered.

We pulled the gurney from the ambulance and wheeled Joe in. One of the nurses took report from us, eyeing Joe sideways. Joe watched them all closely, and before I left, I turned to him and ordered him to behave himself. He patted my hand and smiled, his head falling back on the hospital pillow for a needed rest. I hoped he would be treated with the respect he deserved and not with the respect he was currently earning.

With clean sheets on the gurney, my partner and I headed for the back doors. My partner still had a grin on his face, and I asked him what was wrong.

"Oh, nothing," he replied. "But you know I'll never be able to go to a baseball game again without thinking of Joe." His eyes dropped down, and he smiled sadly as we put the gurney back in the ambulance in preparation for another call.

CHALLENGES

Human beings are designed to take a lot of abuse—physical as well as mental. But sometimes it gets to be too much. I'm sure that somewhere, some psychologist could interview Joe and find a dozen reasons why he was predestined to react to life the way that he did. He claimed to be a Viet Nam Veteran, and I believed him. There were many who came home from that war and were not able to cope with what they saw or did and ended up just dropping out.

One of the biggest challenges of working in an area like this and dealing with people every day is to avoid judging them based on the standards of the rest of society. I used to volunteer to work in the worst areas of town because I found it humbling—because it reminded me that there, but for the grace of God, was I or someone in my family. The medics, firefighters, and police officers who I had the most respect for were the ones who could work this awful area of town day after day and still call these people sir or madam; they deserve that. It's an old cliché, but one that needs repeating often when dealing with other people: "Never judge a man until you have walked a mile in his moccasins."

I have been witness to, and occasionally victim to, disrespect from people in all areas of medicine, but for some reason it is rampant in emergency areas. My husband and I once had a family friend prejudged by staff in a hospital as being crazy and in withdrawal because he tested positive for marijuana in his urine. He was, in fact, a cancer patient who used marijuana medicinally for pain and appetite. He was confused not due to withdrawal or intoxication but because his blood sodium levels were so low they threatened his life. Both of us being professionals at the hospital in question, we were able to rectify most of the problematic judgment simply by identifying him as a friend of ours and speaking directly, and professionally, to the doctors and nurses in charge of his case. I hate to think what could have happened to our friend had we not been able to play the nurse/doctor card.

But I have also been witness to wonderful forms of grace in some of the people who worked in those areas. Nurses who wouldn't discharge people like Joe until they had fed him a hot meal. X-ray techs taking up a collection for a cab to the shelter for a homeless mom. Nurses' aides shopping thrift stores for sweat suits so people could have a clean change of clothes to wear home.

Life hands all of us challenges. Some, for whatever reason, can't cope with those challenges. And I think we all probably have a breaking point.

IT'S ALL ABOUT THE TEAM

There are areas of every town that attract the members of society whose existence most of us choose to deny in our regular lives. Yet there were those of us that worked in the field of emergency medicine who liked working in these areas. For me it was the need of the people who lived there. When we were called out down there, it was usually for someone who really had a medical problem that needed to be addressed. The majority of the population in this area didn't have any medical coverage at all—not even the state-issued medical coverage for low-income people. You had to have an address and tenacity in order to be granted coverage, and this population was either transient or had somehow lost the drive required to deal with government programs and their required paperwork.

We were responding to an address just a few blocks from our station. The dispatcher had announced it was for a male of unknown age who was not breathing. There was a huge population of drug abusers in this area with heroin being the drug of choice. Overdoses were common enough that we had a protocol that allowed us to treat a heroin overdose with a direct IV push of Narcan, the medication that worked as an antidote for heroin and restored the respiratory drive of someone who had overdosed within just a few seconds if we gave it in time. This protocol had been implemented as a response to the number of overdose patients who would wake up after an IV was established and Narcan given—only to walk off down the street dragging the IV after them for fear of legal repercussions. This call was to an apartment building that was notorious for these calls.

Pulling up in front of the apartment building, we grabbed the gear from the back of the ambulance and headed up the stairs to the apartment we had been dispatched to. I was in front carrying my twelve-lead EKG monitor and the drug box. My partner, Scott, followed with the respiratory bag.

This was the first time I had ever worked with Scott. He had worked as a volunteer firefighter for many years, so I had confidence in his skills should we have to challenge them. My only concern was that he seemed a bit naïve to the workings of humanity in the big city. I too had come from a background in which the happenings in the big city were a foreign concept. Scott would learn the same way the rest of us did, especially if he kept working in this district.

The door to the apartment we had been sent to was standing wide open, and there was no one around. Stopping just outside the door, I yelled inside, "Hello, anyone in there?" Scott, still feeling the adrenaline rush of a newbie, rushed past me and into the apartment. "Scott, slow down." His adrenaline had taken hold, and he had tunnel vision on the crumpled body on the far side of the room that was sitting on the floor half propped against the wall. Glancing down, I saw the trail of used hypodermics that indicated this was a crash pad. Junkies would use one apartment to shoot up and sleep off the initial drowse before going out into the world to do whatever it was that junkies did to get their money for the drugs.

"Damn it, Scott. *Stop!*" I ordered. He had not seen those needles, and I was afraid he would step on something or worse—kneel on one. Fortunately the training for volunteers was fairly rigorous and very militaristic. At my order Scott froze next to the man on the floor and looked my way. "Look down, Scott," I said, indicating the littered floor. "Nasty needles, partner. Watch yourself." Glancing down, Scott's eyes widened. He looked back up at me and nodded his thanks. "He's probably hot too," I said, tilting my head at our patient and using the street lingo for people with dirty needles in their pockets or flesh.

Using more caution now, Scott dropped to one knee beside the man on the floor. Still a little too excited for my taste, he reached out for a pulse, knocking the man sideways. I didn't have to feel for a pulse as the man fell but didn't unbend from his half sitting position. "Scott, stop." I said quietly.

Scott's adrenaline was pumping back up as he began ripping open the respiratory bag. "He's not breathing!" he yelled at me.

Stepping forward between Scott and the equipment he was about to violate, I laid a hand firmly on his shoulder. "Scott, stop. This guy is not going to breathe again. Take a deep breath yourself and look again." I said gently.

Anger flashed across Scott's face, but he did as he had been told. He took a deep breath and then really looked. The man was wearing only a pair of soiled boxer shorts, and his age was indeterminable. Not only was the pallor of death distorting his face, but he was obviously a hard-core junkie, judging by the easily visible track-mark bruises traveling up both arms. Junkies lived a hard life, and whatever damage wasn't done to them by the drugs was accomplished by a lifestyle of always looking for that next fix. Rigor mortis had taken a firm hold of the remains of this man. Gravitational pooling of blood called lividity had left vivid purple and blue marks on the backs of the man's legs and buttocks. They were now readily visible as he lay on his side awkwardly frozen in the semisitting position into which he had tipped because of Scott's rush to help.

"Shit," said Scott. His shoulders slumped as the realization hit him. Looking up at me, he asked, "Well, now what?"

I had already pulled my fire-department portable radio from the holster on my hip. Clicking the repeater button and attempting to call dispatch only brought me the static of a weak signal. There were radio towers in the area, and if the battery in the portable was starting to go weak, they would occasionally block transmission. "Now we wait for the coroner," I said to Scott as I stepped back around the side of the wall the man had been sitting against and tried my radio again. Rewarded by the all-business sound of the dispatcher's voice, I cancelled the approaching engine and asked her to send the coroner to our location. Stepping back around the wall, I bent to examine the deceased man a little more closely.

"Fix him." A shadow brushed over my back as the shaky voice grabbed my attention.

Whirling around, I was horrified to find my partner gone with most of the equipment and a thin, wobbly man with a scraggly beard standing in the doorway. One hand held him steady in the door; the other held a six-inch knife. The only thing left for me to grab was the EKG monitor, and I grasped it by the handle, pulling it around in front of me. "Was this gentleman a friend of yours?" I upbraided myself for not making sure my partner knew the team rules in this area: first and foremost never leave your partner alone! Jabbing the knife in the air in front of him, the man made it clear he was not open for conversation. "I said fix him!" he growled.

Stepping back to put myself in the doorway to the other room, I kept my monitor firmly held in front of me. "Listen, your friend has been dead awhile." Hoping this one wasn't too stoned to understand, I tried reason. "There's not anything we can do at this point."

The shadow in the doorway advanced two steps, still jabbing with the knife. "I said fix him!" he ordered, getting more agitated. "You've got the magic drug; now fix him."

There was nothing I was going to be able to do for his friend, but I put my hand in my jumpsuit pocket in an attempt to stall. Empty. I almost always carried two preloaded syringes of Narcan, the antidote for heroin, in my pocket in this area, yet for some reason this morning, I had neglected to put them there. "Look," I said, trying to reason once again, "I would help him if I could. I can't. He's been gone too long."

"Listen, bitch," the shadowed man growled at me, "quit making excuses, and fix him." He moved closer, still waving the knife in the air in front of him. I pulled the EKG monitor hard against my chest. Thoughts of my family scurried through my head, my heart pounding in my chest. I had been in many physical encounters before but never completely alone.

Adrenaline is triggered in stressful situations as part of the fight-or-flight response that helped us evolve so successfully, but it also causes huge problems in people assaulted by horrific emotions in emergencies. Emergency responders learn early on to control this flightiness caused by pumping hormones and to direct it to reason. There is also a level of tolerance we develop for the natural drug. This man had neither reason nor tolerance, and while I understood his response to his friend's death, I also knew this was a horribly dangerous position for me to be in. The visible track marks on his arms registered as I tried again. "I need you to back off," I said as firmly as I could.

"Fuck you," he countered and began advancing with the knife in front of him.

I pulled back on the handle of my monitor, preparing to use it to fight with. Not the perfect weapon, but it was heavy and would hurt. He was obviously stoned and so much slower than I was, but he was also heavily medicated so he wouldn't feel the pain of the fight either.

"Jack, what the fuck?" Another voice in the doorway. My aggressor spun around to face the door. Outlined there was a heavy man bent with age. "What the fuck are you doin', man?"

Jack suddenly shrank. Losing his doped-out, violent intentions, he simply folded in on himself. "Oh, man," he began to mumble as rapidly as a child makes excuses to an elder. "We shot up together. He was alive, man. It was good stuff, man. We were going to dose then go to the docks and bum some change. Dude, I couldn't wake him up! He's all hard, and I couldn't wake him up, man. She won't fix him." He sobbed into the other man's arms.

The man surveyed the scene silently over Jack's head. "Give me the knife, and get the fuck outta here 'fore the cops come," he said.

Jack, suddenly tired and weak, handed his weapon over to the new guy and meekly faded out the door.

"Thanks," I managed through my dry mouth.

"Yeah," said my rescuer, "don't they teach you idiots anything? If I hadn't come along, he might as well have killed you and never thought about it again."

Drawing a deep breath, I held my tongue as I watched my partner's face go white in shock at the man's words. He had come back up just in time to witness the conclusion of the little drama. He stood speechless as my rescuer folded the knife back into itself and slipped it into his pocket. Looking me up and down and then back at my white-faced partner, he smirked. "Idiots," he murmured again. Then he waved in the police officer who had arrived with the coroner. "Officer Anderson," he said, "another one offed himself. Man, I'm going to have to hire a security guard," he chortled. The smile disappeared from his face as he looked at me sideways. "Don't know who he is. Must have broken in here. He must have been one of those vagrants." We both knew the officer wouldn't believe him, but we also both knew that the man on the floor was long gone.

"Officers." I greeted the men arriving with the black-draped gurney. "No ID. He's been down awhile. Looks like they've been using this place a lot lately," I said, indicating the floor. "I'll file a report with my company for you guys. Watch yourselves." Still holding my monitor by the handle, I led my now very sheepish partner back out to the rig.

"Holy crap, I'm *so* sorry," he started.

Suddenly I felt very tired. "Scott, lesson one in this town: never, ever for whatever reason leave your partner. And I don't want to talk about this anymore," I said as I picked up the mic and cleared us from the scene: ready for another call.

QUEEN TAKES ROOK

I t was a small town nestled up in the foothills. The station was a refurbished mobile home with two bedrooms and two baths tucked onto a hill on the edge of town.

It had been a busy shift for this area, and we hadn't spent much time in quarters. Of course, a busy shift in this town was anything more than two calls in twenty-four hours. Transport times extended from twenty minutes to the local hospital up to three hours for transfers such as the one we were just returning from. The local hospital had basic services but no specialists, and anyone requiring more than standard care usually was loaded into an ambulance from the emergency room and shipped to one of the bigger cities in the area.

We were just outside of the county line from one such transfer when the radio dispatcher asked if we were available for a call to the "Castle." The Castle was a turn-of-the-century school building built of brick made in the local area. It did resemble a castle from the outside, with parapets along the roof and three-story walls with few windows. It dwarfed the rest of the buildings in this quaint little remnant of a mining town.

My partner rolled his eyes at me as I jumped at the chance to see the inside of the building. After its role as a residential school, it had served several different purposes before becoming a halfway house for model prisoners—whatever that meant. I loved old architecture, and sometimes this job let us see inside places the general public only dreamt of seeing.

"Medic one is available for response," I said, letting her know where we were. The second ambulance in the county was also out on a call, leaving only a rig that was up in the high country. It would take them thirty minutes to get to our little town, and we were only twenty minutes away.

"Ten-four, medic one. Code three for a fifty-year-old male with chest pains. See the guard outside the kitchen." My partner lit up the lights, and we headed for the Castle, judiciously using the siren only when we came upon other vehicles—as the veterans in this business we were. Pulling into the gates surrounding the Castle, we were directed by one of the local firefighters up a ramp marked For Deliveries Only. Another firefighter stood at the outside door waiting to direct us in. Grabbing the obligatory EKG monitor and slinging the respiratory bag over my shoulder, I headed up the narrow brick stairway.

"This guy doesn't look too good." The firefighter greeted us. "But he is refusing treatment. Says he wants to go to his own doctor in the morning."

"No problem," I said. "Let's have a look, and if he's O.K., I'm good with that." Turning to my partner, who was following with the drug box at the bottom of the stairs, I said, "Hey, Roger, will you grab the clipboard, please. They say this guy wants to AMA."

An AMA is a document signed by people who have called or had someone call for an ambulance or sought medical care and then changed their minds. It stood for *against medical advice* and basically warned signers that by refusing service, they were going against medical advice and releasing us from any liability for their medical care. Most of the persons we responded to up here had a legitimate medical concern, and sometimes this paper was what it took to get them to actually seek medical care.

Walking through the door behind the firefighter, I was struck by the incredible arched ceiling of this, the most utilitarian of the rooms in this castle. I would love to have seen the rest of it, but given that I now found an obviously sick, middle-aged man lying on the floor of the commercial kitchen, that wasn't going to happen.

Approaching the man, I knelt beside him and introduced myself.

"I'm not going to any fucking hospital!" he said.

"O.K. Once again, I am a paramedic, and we are here because you are having chest pains. The staff called us. We didn't just show up," I tried again.

"Well...I...didn't fuckin' call you! And I'm not goin'. I'm fuckin' fine!" My patient formed his words carefully, but I noticed he did not try to get up, and his pale gray-blue skin tone had no reddish over-tones as he attempted to set me straight.

"Dude! You fuckin' fell out, man!" Wearing a blue uniform, the man who spoke was thin and dark skinned. "You fuckin' turned fuck-in' blue, man."

O.K., not the most eloquent of conversationalists I had heard late-ly, but my patient was listening to him.

"Dude! Man! You fuckin' freaked me out, man!" As he approached, one of the guards in the kitchen stepped forward to block his move-ment. Seeing an unwitting ally here, I waved the guard back.

"Listen to your friend, man. He is really worried." The man sur-veyed my face carefully. His eyes then roved to the surrounding faces and stopped on his friend.

"Awww...fuck you too, man," he said to his partner. "I ain't goin' to no fuckin' hospital!" He sighed deeply as he laid his head back on the floor. His coloring maintained the same grayish-blue shades he'd had when we came in, and with the exertion of his argument, he had developed a sweaty sheen.

"O.K., listen to me, please." I used my tough-guy voice, success-fully diverting his attention from his friend and back to me. "We take your blood pressure, do an EKG, then I'll listen to you." I mo-tioned my partner into the drama. He dropped to his knee and pulled the blood-pressure cuff out of the respiratory bag, wrapping it around the guy's arm. *Dude*, as he had become in my mind since no one—including himself—had given me any other name to address him by, started to object. I countered any and all objections by pulling his shirt apart and began the application of electrodes, which I would plug into the EKG machine.

An EKG showed only the electrical activity of the heart, but since any disruption in the mechanical workings of the heart or the oxygen flow to it affected how the electricity was conducted, it would show me some of what I needed to know.

As I expected, dude responded to my activity with the electrodes negatively, but it was distracting him from my partner. "Seventy over thirty," my partner said. "Checked it twice."

Dude's angry look and his objections to my application of the electrodes were interrupted by the tone in my partner's voice. "What the fuck does that mean?" he demanded, "Seventy over thirty."

"It's not good, man," my partner said, holding dude's attention as I flipped on my monitor.

The EKG fuzzed in, showing me a rhythm that made *my* heart beat faster. Dude had what is called in the field "tombstone T-waves." It meant that the ventricles in his heart were trying to recharge the electricity, which causes the heart to pump blood, at the same time that they were sending the current to cause a second beat. This would cause the heart muscle to become confused and unable to pump the blood that kept him alive. Dude was in serious danger here. In the meantime, he was busy assuring my partner that his parentage was less then desirable.

"Dude," I said, trying to again gain his attention, "I just hooked you up to the EKG, and it is not good."

"Fuck you."

O.K., I had his attention. "Listen to me. You are having a heart attack."

"Yeah, right. Fuck you." An interesting exchange, but not very rewarding in its variety of nouns and verbs. "I am still *not* going to the fuckin' hospital, and you can't make me." Dude concluded the conversation in his eloquent style.

Sitting back on my heels, I looked at my patient. He knew what was happening and was still refusing treatment. One more try. "Do you understand that you are going to die?" I asked. Not the time to pull punches, I continued. "Are you ready to die, dude? 'Cause it is going to happen really soon if you don't go to the hospital."

"Fuckin' 'stablishment! I ain't buyin'. *And* I ain't goin' to no hospital."

Still sitting back, I looked at my patient. I had no doubt in my mind that this man was having a massive heart attack and that he would indeed die very soon without help. However, to take him to the hospital without his consent was kidnapping, and I was not ready to go to jail for this guy. But I was not going to lose my job over him, either.

"O.K. All right. Then I've got to call the doctor I work for first," I explained. "I can't leave you here without talking to him because you are going to die right here and right now, and I am not going to get fired because you are so damn pig headed."

I looked him straight in the eye. Dude looked me up and down and snorted. He had to feel like crap. His heart was dying, and he still just didn't get it. I had no idea how else to get through to him.

Standing up, I left the EKG electrodes on his chest. I pulled my radio from its holster and tried to contact the hospital. Static was all I was getting. "That won't work in here." One of the guards spoke the obvious and then added reason to his statement. "Too much rebar in these walls. Signal can't get out."

"Great place to have a halfway house," I thought as I headed for the door. Hopefully I would be able to reach the hospital from the porch, as the repeaters for the radio were in a direct line from there.

I had to go halfway down the stairs before I got a signal. Calling the base hospital, I asked to speak to the doctor on duty. I had to wait a few minutes as the nurse went to fetch the physician who she had said was "in with a patient."

"Tombstone T-waves, cool, pale, diaphoretic. BP of seventy, systolic. This guy is on his way out and refusing care." I let the doctor know what I was up against. "No radio inside, or I would have you talk to him." Sometimes that helped. *Doctor* was still a magic word to most people, and they wouldn't argue with one the way they would with us.

I was finishing up my radio presentation as the door above me slammed open. "Hey! You need to get back in here!" the firefighter shouted. "He's out again, and your monitor has gone haywire."

The doctor was talking as I switched off my radio and ran back up the stairs. Looking down from the inside stairs, I saw that my patient was indeed out again. He was not breathing and was turning blue. Running down the stairs, I looked at my monitor and was not surprised to see ventricular fibrillation, a rhythm in which the ventricles of the heart were in a nonrhythmic quiver as opposed to a steady beat. It would not pump blood like this.

Grabbing the paddles off my monitor, I quickly checked that the leads were still attached. My partner was ready with the conduction gel. Squeezing a glob on one paddle, I rubbed the two together briskly and then applied them to my patient's chest. I leaned forward so that the pressure of my weight would assure that the electricity I was about to apply would go through the heart and hopefully stop it. This would allow the natural electrical rhythm to reset itself, kind of like rebooting a computer. "Clear!" I yelled over the escalating whine of the charging monitor. *Beep, beep, beep.* It made its readiness known as I pushed down on the red discharge buttons with my hands. The electricity coursing through the man's body made his body jump.

"Fuck! That fuckin' hurt!" The previously unconscious and nonbreathing man's response to the electrical shock threw me briefly as he reached up and clutched at his chest. His eyes opened slowly, and he looked straight into my eyes. Adrenaline still flowing, I held out my paddles to show the man. "Dying hurts, dude! Are you ready to go now, or do I do this again?"

Still rubbing his chest, my patient's face showed horror as I held out the paddles. "No...Fuck, no..." he said, quiet now. "Don't fuckin' do that anymore! I'll go."

Waving to my partner, I left him and the firefighters in charge of getting the gurney as I held my paddles over my resistant patient. The paddles didn't return home until my patient, my partner, and I were loaded in the ambulance and well on our way to the hospital.

"Do you fuckin' do that to everyone that doesn't want to go to the hospital?" my patient asked.

"Only the ornery ones," I said. "Only the ornery ones."

FEAR

In our society with its fast pace and competitive edge, there seems to be a pervasive undercurrent. Having witnessed the moments of life that cause the façade to drop, I can name the current. It is fear. Fear of the loss of control, fear of failure, fear of dying, fear of self, fear of others—the fears are too innumerable to count. Nevertheless, they are there, and they persist. I used to think that the fear was spawned by our societal way of life: the fast pace, keeping up with the Joneses. Then I realized that the fear exists even in those who claim to have escaped the mainstream of society. From those rich enough to buy an analyst for every occasion and the homeless souls who live in cardboard boxes to the newly arrived immigrants who have yet to learn the American way of life, the fears are the same. I have begun to believe that the underlying fears are what make humans the evolutionary success story that we are. We are so afraid of failing, dying, or being laughed at that we forget to let ourselves enjoy life, and yet we need to be afraid, to worry in order to maintain life. It creates an interesting paradox of survival.

There have been a few times in my life when I have not been afraid. I was not afraid at those times when adrenaline was pumping so exquisitely through my veins that my senses were numbed to any examination of self-preservation. And when I have been alone—so completely alone—that the consequences of the realization of the fears did not matter.

I once asked a homeless man, "Why?" He was sober. He was sick. He was afraid. So in the safe harbor that was the back of my ambulance, I asked him why he was homeless. He told me in a rational manner that indeed it was his choice. He told me that fear of life made him homeless. He didn't have to worry about losing his home or his wife or his status. In addition, he rationalized with great clarity that this was the resolution of difficulties that had seen him arrive at his current state. Yet as he spoke, the fear spilled out around him. He had no home to lose, but another homeless person had stolen his cardboard box. Was I sure that the police officer that had been with us on scene had taken care of his shopping cart? Did County Hospital feed you before they let you go? Could I make sure they gave him a sandwich? He had abandoned life for fear of losing what could have been and now feared losing only what existed in the immediate. His fears were the same as the mother of the man who owned half the county. She lived in an expansive apartment decorated exquisitely with imported antiques. She had servants to care for her and her surroundings. Yet she worried about the dinner she had left on the table being ruined. Was I sure her maid had secured the house prior to her leaving? Did I think the hospital would let her have something to eat? Maybe just a sandwich?

I wish I could say that my exposure to the phenomenon of eminent fear had cured me of worry. It hasn't. When I watch my dog hide his bone from the other dogs in the pack, I think that maybe being a little afraid is just part of being alive. Maybe all the self-help books, medications, and TV shows that teach us how not to fear haven't accepted that we have to worry about that sandwich to survive.

"OH MY GOD, LUCILLE"

S he had come by the station early in the day. Having just signed up at the volunteer fire department, she was young, excited, a little extreme in her desire to save humanity, and she *really* wanted to be a paramedic like on TV. "That is my life's goal!" She informed us with the breathless wonder of a contestant in the Miss USA pageant. Always eager to help out people who were interested in examining the realm of our chosen profession, we had asked her in, shown her the ambulance, and talked to her about her aspirations and where she could go for the training she would need. Sheila, as she introduced herself, had shown up with the required paperwork to do a ride along, a chance for those who were interested in this career to experience life as we saw it. I liked her enthusiasm and agreed to let her ride with us. Several hours of her perkiness, however, sent me to my room with a headache. Roger, my EMT partner, reveled in the glow of her adoration at his being "a *real* EMT" and had kept her entertained all morning with his limited collection of war stories.

The first call we'd been sent out on was a very minor traffic accident, where our little volunteer took blood pressures on both the people involved with the adrenaline rush that only the rookies remember. It had been a fender bender, and neither party was hurt, both refusing treatment and transport. You could see the look of disappointment cross her face when my partner took out the clip-board to have both people sign the AMA forms that would release us from liability if they should later decide they really were hurt after all.

Returning to quarters, she bounced with excitement when my partner announced he was going to wash the rig. I let them have at it and used the opportunity to fix some lunch and catch the noon news. Sheila was still trotting along behind my partner like an excit-able new puppy when they came back inside, and I could tell her en-thusiasm was even beginning to wear a little thin on Roger—in spite of his maleness. I escaped the necessity of again retiring to my room as the dispatch phone rang. This station was located in an area that made radio contact iffy at best, so we were dispatched by telephone. Grabbing the phone before I could, my partner wrote down the ad-dress while Sheila clapped her hands in excitement. "Chest pain," he said as he headed toward the door. "Eighty-six-year-old female."

I turned and watched as he tucked happy Sheila in the back and made sure she had fastened her seat belt. I wasn't sure it would hold her enthusiasm in as we headed out code three, Sheila talking all the while. The call wasn't far—just across town—and neither Roger nor I said a word. Pulling up in front of the address given, I grabbed my monitor and, letting Sheila out, handed her the respiratory bag. She grinned ear to ear at me, and then as she looked up, the smile was gone, and her eyes popped into that deer-in-the-headlights look. Roger reached around and grabbed the drug box. "What's up, Sheila?" he asked, seeing the look on her face.

"That's Lucille's house," she said slowly. "I didn't know we were coming here."

"Neither did we," joked Roger.

"Is there a problem?" I asked as I walked up the steps. Better to know before we went inside.

"She goes to my church. She's like a grandma to me," said Sheila as she reapplied the smiley face, although it remained slightly askew.

"You O.K.?" Roger asked over his shoulder.

Sheila ran to catch up. "Sure." It was obviously a little forced, but we all had to learn sometime that this job—this life—was not a cool TV show. It was reality.

The house was an eloquently appointed Victorian with gingerbread accoutrements and furnishings to match. Our patient, in fact, matched the house in her dress and demeanor, reclining on a fainting couch with her worried daughter in attendance. Lucille was indeed a gentlewoman as she welcomed us into her home and apologized for not getting up. Her pale face and the beading sweat of her brow, which she kept dabbing at with her lace-trimmed hanky, sparked my concern.

As I knelt beside our patient and began to ask her questions, her eyes rested on Sheila, whom had faded to the back. "Why, Sheila darling, I didn't know you were working on the ambulance?"

Sheila blushed but seemed to perk at the recognition. "I'm going to go to school to be an EMT!" she explained to the reclining Lucille. Roger took the opportunity to open the respiratory bag and hand Sheila the blood pressure cuff and stethoscope as he pulled a nasal cannula out and applied it to Lucille's delicate face. "Just a little oxygen, ma'am," he explained.

Repetition was key in learning emergency medicine. When overwhelmed by stressful situations or horrifying distractions, repetition in learning meant that the hands would know what to do while the head caught up with what was going on. Sheila had obviously been practicing her blood pressure methods as her hands readily performed the required task, allowing my partner and me to begin the more advanced care.

Covering Lucille with a throw from the couch, I reached under and undid her high-necked dress and bra. Years of experience let me apply the electrodes where they needed to go without exposing Lucille to undo embarrassment.

The volunteer fire department members had pulled in behind us, removed the gurney from the ambulance, and were setting it up for Lucille as I switched on my monitor. It was a disorganized rhythm known as atrial fibrillation. A-fib for short, it means that the smaller chambers in the heart, the atria, were no longer beating in an organized rhythm. Many people live years with this heart rhythm, but Lucille denied having any cardiac history at all, and as I watched the paper strip march out, on the monitor I saw an additional fluctuation known as rapid ventricular response, which concerned me. This pattern meant that Lucille's heart was being irritated by whatever was causing the new disorganized beat. Working quickly now, I started an IV and had the firefighters lift Lucille onto the gurney. She was still complaining of chest pain, but her blood pressure was only eighty over sixty, which made it impossible for me to administer nitroglycerin or morphine as both could cause her blood pressure to drop even further.

The fire department worked well as a team, and Sheila was in her moment rechecking the blood pressure every five minutes for me. I was glad to have her along for the ride.

As the team loaded Lucille and all of my gear in the back of the ambulance, I took the opportunity to call the base hospital. I was not happy when one of my least favorite nurses answered the radio. Most hospitals mandated extensive training for the registered nurses who were allowed to answer the radios when the ambulances called. We worked under protocols that covered pretty much anything we could do in the field, but we still had to call the hospital to O.K. the protocol we were following. It could then approve or reject the choice of the paramedic for treatment the patient was receiving. Most of the time the hospitals trusted the judgments of the field crews, as we could see the patient and they could not. This specific nurse however had earned a reputation for arguing, usually inappropriately, with the paramedics in the field ever since her ugly divorce from one of the medics the year before. She always seemed to divert back to a protocol that call for albuterol, a drug used for asthma. The brand name was Proventil, and her nick-name had become Patty Proventil because she ordered it so often.

I had a bad feeling about what was to come as I made my initial radio presentation to Patty Proventil, and true to form, she directed me to deviate from my chosen treatment route and give the patient albuterol. I argued with her that the patient's heart was already irritated and that I was afraid we would complicate matters further. She came back on by saying that she was familiar with this patient and the doctor was standing by the radio and agreed with her directions. To refuse the order now that the base physician was involved could cause serious problems for me and the company I was working for, should I be wrong.

"Patty?" was all Roger said as he arched his eyebrows when I told him to set me up an albuterol treatment before we left scene. I didn't need to affirm and sat my monitor in the jump seat where I could watch it. Sheila climbed in behind me and promptly started taking another blood pressure. Roger looked at Sheila, his infatuation gone, rolled his eyes at me, and headed for the driver's seat.

I took the drive time to quickly go through the cornucopia of herbal medications and doctor-issued drugs that Lucille kept in a shoebox, writing them down on paperwork. Glancing up at the monitor, I was horrified to see Lucille's heart rhythm go from A-Fib to a deadly rhythm known as supraventricular tachycardia, or SVT for short. Lucille's heart was pumping at close to two hundred beats a minute, which was too fast to allow it to refill between beats. Lucille slumped back in the seat, and her hand dropped the nebulizer she had been holding to her mouth. "Oh my God, Lucille!" screamed Sheila at the sight of her friend fading away. Reaching for the paddles on the monitor, I was shocked to see a slight pause and then the resumption of a normal sinus rhythm on my monitor. Feeling for a pulse, I was thrilled that it corresponded. Lucille lifted her head and reached to rub her eyes.

Sheila sat behind me as pale as Lucille with her eyes and mouth both wide open. Reassured by Lucille's now strong pulse and the corresponding beat on the monitor, I turned my attention to Sheila.

Sheila's eyes were not leaving the monitor. I patted her hand. "She's going to be—" was all I got out before Sheila's eyes again grew huge. Turning my attention back to the monitor, I was horrified to see an even more deadly rhythm march across the green and gray screen: ventricular tachycardia. Lucille's eyes again rolled back as her head slumped to the side.

"Oh my God, Lucille!" again echoed through my tiny compartment, and again the rhythm on the monitor stalled and then resumed a nice, normal, healthy-looking sinus beat.

"What the hell is going on back there?" Roger yelled, looking briefly in the rearview mirror. "Nothing I can't handle yet," I said, leaving my response open for an addendum.

Lucille had picked her head back up and was staring at Sheila, who in turn was fixated on the monitor. Sheila's eyes again dilated, and I looked quickly to the monitor. The SVT had returned in force at over two hundred this time. Lucille again slumped in her seat, and I again reached toward the monitor. "Oh my God, Lucille!" Again, my partner swerved just slightly, and Lucille's heart began to convert itself to what in any other circumstance would be considered normal. Lucille again opened her eyes, and stared at Sheila. Grabbing the blood pressure cuff off the floor where it had fallen, I reached out to check my patient's pulse. Good and strong. Lucille diverted her gaze from Sheila to me. "Is everything O.K.?" she asked in her genteel voice, and then her head dropped again. Looking over at the monitor, I was horrified to see ventricular fibrillation, the most deadly of rhythms.

"Oh my God, Lucille!" emanated from behind me, and I watched as the monitor changed its course and looked normal. It was an unusual treatment, but it appeared to be working. I reached up to my medication cabinet for a drug called lidocaine, which would stop the irritation that was going on in the heart. Lucille was looking a little tired now as she kept her head back on the gurney and looked at Sheila. "Honey, are you sure you want to do this?" said Lucille as Sheila continued her wide-eyed staring contest with the monitor.

I uncapped the lid to the drug and attached the plunger. "Oh my God, Lucille!"

Another run of ventricular tachycardia. It was like a horror code from an advanced-life-support class where students were taught how to deal with cardiac emergencies. And with Sheila's scream, Lucille was back. Attaching the syringe to the flowing IV, I gave Lucille half a dose of the drug because of her age and her home medications. Lucille sat back drowsily for the remaining two or three minutes of our ride. Sheila was fixated on the monitor; I didn't try to distract her. She was proving quite helpful.

Feeling a bit irritated, I was rather short in my report to the doctor. Sheila called her mother for a ride home from the hospital and left the fire department. I heard she went away to college. I doubt she went into medicine.

DENIAL

People almost always have the need to see what happened to the other guy, hence our compulsion to stare when we drive past traffic accidents or scenes where there are ambulances and fire trucks. The television news lately seems completely devoted to this aspect of human nature. There is a profound and compulsive need to know the worst that happened to the other guy, whether it is a tragedy that is newsworthy or a life that commands a reality show of its own. We as a society have sunk to such a level of macabre interest that the media is inundated with reality shows in which trauma happens—but only in a controlled and survivable manner. And, of course, always to the other guy.

In addition, the evolving society in which we exist is becoming more violent and threatening us on a personal level almost daily. Mass killings by strangers in random settings, terrorist attacks, and kidnappings have all become an inescapable part of our everyday existence. In addition, the more transparent our lives are, the less denial we can wrap around ourselves, and the more neurotic we become. As a society and as individuals we are trapped in a reality that has disintegrated with the modern media into a world in which the requisite level of denial for living is absent. Mass communication has made what used to be a shadow of our worst fears now a taunting mask at the window that can no longer be ignored.

Emergency medical workers have always lived somewhere on the edge of this shadow land, seeing and treating the truth of the ugly side of life. Lessons should be learned from these professionals. One of the most telling personality traits in determining the career length of an emergency care worker is the ability to separate the self from the reality of what we see and treat every day. Compartmentalization of events and self is paramount in the ability to function at peak capacity during times of stress or ongoing trauma. Believing *it* can happen to us or ours while dealing with *it* for someone else is crippling in the most profound way. A reasonable amount of denial that the insanity can affect our families or us is paramount to a happy life.

How impossible it would be to get up every morning with the awareness of the vulnerability of the human condition at the forefront of our minds. To cognitively recognize what would happen if we slipped in the shower or the hair dryer fell in while we splashed water on our face. To have a conscious reality of the dangers of a flash fire when we turn on the stove or the incredible risk we take to drive a vehicle or what would happen to our body if we somehow slipped in the rain and fell *just so*. To spend our working hours answering cries for help from people who have had their denial stripped from them is to live with an extra layer of protection from the pain and the pleasures of life.

When the lines do get crossed by the intrusion of reality into our world of separation, it creates real fear and the type of stress that can end careers or stop them from happening in the first place.

IT WAS THE LEGS

I'd been working with Dave for well over a year. We worked well together. He could guess what I was going to need and have it waiting before I asked. We were good at station life too, as he liked his privacy as much as I did. Although we had become friends, we pretty much kept to ourselves around quarters.

It was late in the day, and we were settling in for what we silently hoped would be a quiet night. The word *quiet* was never spoken out loud around quarters because of the superstition that if it were said, the opposite would happen. So we just sprawled on the couch and hoped.

That hope lasted for about thirty minutes before the lights flashed on and the tones vibrated the speakers in this old house we called home while at work.

"Woman in labor. Water has broken."

Dave and I looked at each other and bent to pull our black work boots on.

I hated driving and was good at maps so that was the way we ran. Pulling the electric line that kept the unit charged when parked at quarters, Dave jumped in the driver's seat while I ran around to the passenger side. Dave waved away the map books as I pulled them from the file on the floor. "I've got it." We had worked this station for a long time, and my partner knew the town very well. We each grabbed a mic, one for the company dispatcher and the other for the county fire dispatcher, and let them know we were responding. By company rules we had to be en route within three minutes. We were headed out in about one.

Around the corner and down a main street, we heard the engine pulling up just ahead of us. This engine was still BLS, a designator that stood for the level of medical training of the personnel. BLS meant basic life support with no paramedics. Since all the ambulances in town ran with at least one paramedic, the fire department still ran a few engines that were staffed with firefighters trained as EMTs. It was a good system but one that would be archaic in a few years as the competition for medical dollars came into play and the fire department started training paramedics and staffing competitive ambulances. For now, it worked. This engine company was one of my favorites. They were used to working with me and my partner, and even the sticky calls worked out well.

As a safety measure, the company's engineer always stayed with the engine and the ambulance outside of the calls unless for some reason we needed extra man power. As we pulled up, he waved us in front of the engine. "The guys are inside already."

I grabbed my OB kit and headed for the door. EMTs were trained in delivering babies, but I knew that this crew had that experience at the bottom of their like-to-do list. They preferred fighting the fires and leaving the medical work to us.

Opening the door for me was a man I knew to be Dad just from his nervous disposition. He bounced back and forth between his feet as he directed me down the hallway, where I could see the blue shirts of the firefighters leaning into a doorway. They parted as they heard me approach, and I realized they were all crowding into a small bathroom. There on the toilet with her legs spread wide and a grimace on her face sat the mom.

I bent down in front of her and had just opened my mouth to start asking the pertinent questions when I heard a hollow splash. That was not good! Unceremoniously I pushed her legs wider, and there in the blood-tinged bowl was the baby. "Guys! Get her off the toilet!" I yelled as I reached between her legs and pulled the baby from the water.

With one firefighter on either side of her, they made short work of helping her down off the toilet and onto the floor in front of me where I worked with the baby. Ripping open the OB kit, I grabbed the suction bulb first and cleaned the nose and mouth. The reward was mine when a quiet little whisper of a cry emanated from the tiny baby girl, who was small enough to fit in one hand. I looked up at Mom in surprise. "I'm twenty-seven weeks," she said, tears streaming down her face, "and it's twins. I thought I was constipated." She cried as she grimaced again.

"Don't push. Whatever you do, don't push," I urged. "Breathe with me now." And I led her through the Lamaze breathing to help stop her from pushing until I could take care of the first baby. "Guys, I need the gurney and another kit," I ordered without looking up.

Twenty-seven weeks is a frighteningly early delivery for a child. A baby can survive at that age but only with immediate and specialized care. And she had just said *twins*! Grabbing my fire radio, I switched the channels with one hand and warned the hospital what we were bringing in.

Tossing my radio aside, I quickly clamped the collapsing umbilical cord just as a pair of little feet poked out from Mom. "Guys, I need another kit…Guys?" Glancing over my shoulder, I was horrified to see an empty doorway. My thoughts were quickly directed back to Mom as she moaned loudly. Turning back to her, I wrapped the first baby in a towel to keep it warm and laid it next to her feet. And gently, very gently, I grasped the tiny feet and helped her sister into the world. Feeling a bump on my shoulder, I looked down to see a second OB kit opened and ready lying next to her squirming sister. Relief flooded me as I grabbed the bulb syringe and suctioned a second tiny nose and mouth.

Looking up, I saw Dave leaning against the doorjamb with a very silly grin on his face. "Thought you might need some help," he said.

"The ambulance is full of firefighters. Tell me you didn't send all of them for the gurney?" He definitely had a knack for relieving the tension.

I looked down at Mom, and she was bleeding a little heavily for my comfort. We would be going code three for the babies and Mom. "Dave, get them to set me up two IVs, please," I said.

I had just finished clamping the cord for the second little girl, and I handed Dave both infants wrapped in delivery blankets and towels as two of the firefighters came back in with the gurney. They looked a little sheepish as they helped lift Mom onto the gurney. "It was the feet," the engineer whispered as we hurried out to the waiting ambulance.

The worst threat to a premature infant at this stage was chilling. We had to get them warmed and to a hospital where they could be put in incubators. I quickly tossed my gear in the side door of the ambulance and climbed in the back. There in the jump seat sat Dave, the silly grin still on his face. He held a small bundle in each hand cuddled up against his chest.

"Who's driving?" I asked horrified.

Grinning up at me, Dave answered, "Seems you've traumatized the firefighters with visions of teeny, tiny feet. The engineer is driving us, and the rest will follow in the fire engine." Dave redirected his eyes and efforts to warming and charming the two little girls. I directed my attention to Mom, starting two IVs and padding for the heavy bleeding. Our firefighting engineer handled the ambulance very quickly and smoothly as we wailed through the quiet streets to the hospital where they waited with two incubators and a full staff of neonatal nurses.

Amanda and Amelia both lived, although the one that had landed in the toilet water did have some initial breathing issues. Dave and I went back to the station feeling very full of ourselves and knowing that we would get months of teasing from the firefighters out of this one.

ALWAYS WORSE ON THE OTHER SIDE

It had been an awful shift. We had been up all night running the kinds of calls that paramedics hate to run. In addition to the everyday awfulness, we'd had two codes that we'd fought to keep alive but failed, a very ugly and successful suicide by train, two childbirths, a shooting in retaliation for the stabbing that we'd also taken in, a nasty motor-vehicle accident, and a standby at a house fire where a family didn't make it out in time. We had only been back in quarters since 4:30 a.m. Exhausted but too tired to sleep, we made coffee and packed our gear, anxious to go home to the safety of denial that lived there.

I was just coming back in from my truck when the lights again flashed on and the tones stabbed at us from the walls. "Code three for a male not breathing." Thinking that Grandpa did not make it through the night, I looked at my partner, and with a sigh we both dropped our personal gear and headed for the ambulance.

The address was a straight shot for us. The engine would be coming across town, as the one assigned to our district was still at the house fire. My partner and I were both too tired to talk as we pulled up to the scene. Fortunately we had worked together for a long time, and each knew how the other worked.

Dave was one of my favorite partners. I could trust him to have my back and keep me functioning at peak even when I was tired. We were good together as partners, and if I had to have a shift like this, I was glad it was with Dave.

Stepping out of the ambulance, I was greeted by a screaming woman on the front lawn. "Here, here!" she screeched. Looking across at Dave, I grabbed my respiratory bag and the monitor and headed for the doorway into which she had disappeared. Dave grabbed the drug box and followed.

The apartment was dark and shadowed after the bright light of the morning sun outside. At first I didn't see anyone. Then I noticed the recliner chair facing away from me and the bald head peaking over the top. "Gramps is having a bad morning," Dave whispered to me as we approached the chair. Still a few steps from the chair, the woman from the lawn came flying back down the hallway carrying a bag. Rushing straight for the chair, she grabbed at the bald head we had seen peaking over the top and, still screaming, threw it at me. The respiratory bag and the monitor hit the floor hard as I reflexively reached out to catch. And catch I did. An infant. A very cold and blue infant. Horrified I looked at Dave. Readjusting the drug box into his left hand, he grabbed the monitor and respiratory bag with his right. We made eye contact, and then he nodded at the door. Turning I headed for the door as fast as I could. Dave was talking to the screaming woman in a low voice, calming her down. Heading for the back of the ambulance, my feet slipped in the still dew-wet grass, and I began to slide down the sloped hill of the front lawn. One foot in front and my back leg curled awkwardly under me, I slid down the hill as I struggled not to drop the infant. I came out of my slide in a run and aimed straight for the open back door of my ambulance.

Once inside I had a minute to assess the baby. I was guessing SIDS. An awful joke on the joy of motherhood, it takes young and healthy infants in their sleep with no warning. There was nothing I was going to be able to do for this baby. He was cold to the touch, his tiny arms and legs were stiff, and the pooling of blood after death had left purple and blue marks on the side of his face.

Dave opened the side door of the ambulance. I could still hear him talking in his calm voice to the mother, assuring her that I was a really good medic and that I would do everything I could do for her baby. He looked in at me, and I shook my head in the negative. His eyes blinked in acknowledgement, and he closed the side doors. I heard him open the front passenger door and, still in his calm voice, deposit Mom in the front. He reached across and clipped her seat belt.

I switched over to the jump seat so that my back would block the mother's view of the baby if she thought to look into the back. I could do nothing. This was now Dave's call.

Picking up the fire radio, Dave told the dispatcher to cancel the engine and explained that we would be code three to the closest hospital. He then started talking calmly to Mom, and I listened, getting the information I needed from their conversation.

Switching on the medical radio in the back, I made contact with base station at that hospital. "Healthy three-month-old male. Mom found him this a.m. Rigor mortis and pronounced lividity. We are transporting for Mom. Single mom. She is here by herself. Confirm for help for Mom."

"Base station copies, medic. We will have the chaplain waiting."

Sitting back exhausted, I listened to Dave's soothing voice as he gently set Mom up for what would be the worst day of her life: Letting her know that it might not necessarily end the way she wished.

Dave pulled straight into the ambulance bay instead of backing in. That would allow him to take Mom in before I had to get out with her worst nightmare. He would make sure she had the chaplain with her when she came into the room to be with her baby one last time.

I waited until they were through the doors and then got out with the infant. The hospital had assigned a noncritical room for us, and I took the baby in and laid him on the gurney. Giving report to the nurse, I went to the medic room to type up the report that would be needed for the coroner. Dave brought me coffee and asked if I was O.K. I told him, "Hell no, and don't tell me you are either." He had the glint of a tear in his eye as he mumbled something about cleaning the rig and headed outside.

Finishing my paperwork, I turned it in at the desk and headed for the ambulance myself. All I could think was that I wanted to go home—that I'd had enough. And Mom was standing at the ambulance-bay door waiting for me.

"I wanted you to know how grateful I am for all you did," she said, tears flowing freely down her cheeks.

There are times in this business when you would like to hear thank-you just once; this was not one of them. My throat choked up. I couldn't say anything. I hadn't done anything. Tears filled my own eyes as I reached out to hold her. I'm not sure who needed that hug more.

"PERSONALITIES"

The toll that is taken on the personal lives of the people who choose to work in medicine is quite substantial, although none likes to admit it. I do not have the expertise to determine whether the challenges created are due to the personality that chooses the career or the career that causes the personality changes. Perhaps it is a combination of both, as most things are.

The studies I have read on EMS personalities were specific as to the people attracted to the career, stating they are basically risk takers and tend to be more than a little codependent. Even though I spent the largest span of my life working in emergency medicine and do not find those descriptors very flattering, I have to admit to the truth in them. I do know that it allows for an acceptable expression of some of the more detrimental presentations of these personality types because it allows the expressions to be confined to the professional life. That is not always an easy accomplishment.

I am aware that some of my own personal experiences have allowed me to be present for people in need in a way that is, while not always comfortable for me, comforting for them. I also know that some of the experiences that I have had during my career have made me more appreciative of what I have in my personal life.

Have I always dealt with those work stresses in a healthy manner? Definitely not. After one very traumatic call, I quit my job with both ambulance companies I was working for and moved my life and kids to a small coastal town where I bought a fishing boat and fished professionally for four months. During that time, I used up all of my savings and ended up living in a camper with my kids and working any other job than paramedic. I eventually went back to emergency medicine for financial reasons and learned healthier ways to deal with the negative emotions, including counseling.

There are counseling services available to EMS personnel after specific incidents, and at one point I took the training required to be a debriefer, as they are called. It was an effective approach for immediate stress release in some instances but required staff to be available to attend group meetings to vent. After the bad shifts, most of us just wanted to go home and hug our kids. Very few of us were comfortable sharing those emotions in a group setting.

A very important part of being effective in medicine is appearing to have a calm and in-control manner. That means swallowing the naturally occurring human emotions of fear, anger, horror, disgust, amazement, etc.—basically remaining fully functional while wanting to scream, cry, run, or giggle hysterically. One of my partners used to joke with me that he could judge the severity of the call by how calm I became while talking to patients or their families; the calmer I became, the more concerned he was.

That very trait is what makes it so hard to counsel EMS providers. If they are good at what they do, they simply do not show it while it is happening. They maintain a functional atmosphere in the most emotionally caustic environments imaginable. It is very difficult to suppress that kind of emotion and then openly express it later in a room full of people—even if those people went through the same incident.

I have been fortunate in that my later career landed me in a position of authority in which after a "bad one," I could talk to people quietly and individually. Talking about it is the key to relieving that kind of stress, but most of the personalities I speak of would never let their guard down while working.

Is there a solution? Not a universal one. Having counselors avail-able for emergency medical workers to talk with should they wish, maintaining team spirit, and allowing for ample downtime help. Some of the scars will always remain, but that is because the people who do this job are human like the rest of us.

TRAINING BY THE BAY

He was the captain of his own engine for a large city by the bay. Training all day with the new rookie on the engine had been exhausting but enjoyable. They had been sitting around and eating the gourmet meal that had been prepared by the rookie in an attempt to impress his new company when the tones notified them of a medical call, unknown reason, see the woman at First and Sycamore. Responding code three—unknown was always code three because, well, you ever knew. The engineer handled the engine with the ease of years of experience as he wove in and out of the traffic, blasting through the traffic lights. They beat the ambulance by minutes. Spotting the woman was an easy task as she stood on the corner that they had been dispatched to. She was the only completely naked woman on the corner. In fact she was the only woman on the corner, but then the way she was built and the fact that she was naked negated the existence of any other woman on said corner.

Seeing the lights and hearing the siren animated the naked woman in a way that only a man can appreciate. She started jumping up and down and waving. The waving they could have ignored. The jumping up and down was something they would have encouraged her to continue for a while. Or longer.

Pulling to the curb in front of the waving and bouncing—really bouncing—woman, they disembarked from the engine. The captain had the honor of addressing this fine example of womanhood first. "Evening, ma'am. Did you call 911?" he asked in his most impressively masculine voice.

"Yes, sir," she responded in a voice as musical as the flowing hair that waved around her bare shoulders in the offshore breeze. "It is an emergency, you see," she explained calmly.

"Ah yes," said Captain Randy in his most authoritative voice, "and what is the emergency that you called us for?" The firefighters had all disembarked from the engine and lined up in a row facing the damsel, who in another life could have been—no should have been—a mermaid, with her long, flowing hair and beautiful sea-green eyes.

"Why, it was the bad guys," she said in her lisping voice that hinted of the South and poured through those magnificent, pouty lips as she shared the glory of those green eyes with all four firefighters.

"Oh dear," said Captain Randy in a voice he hoped conveyed his dedication and caring soul. "What bad guys would those be?" He avoided saying dear but only by a breath.

"Why," she said, raising a delicately fingered hand up across her penthouse-perfect chest, "the ones that broke into my house."

"Ah yes," said Randy, as the other firefighters stood mute in the glory of this once-in-a-lifetime experience. "And did they hurt you?" he asked in his most caring voice.

She paused as she contemplated the response. The firefighters could see her assessing each and every one of her body parts mentally. In fact they joined her—mentally of course. "Why, not really," she said in her breathy voice. "Well, only a little. They were actually rather nice." She gazed up at the adoring audience she had obtained.

"And what did they do?" Captain Randy asked as his testosterone flared in defense of this poor, helpless female.

"Why, they broke in my door," she said, her green eyes glowing like emeralds with little diamonds of tears forming in the corners as they grew big with the retelling of her trauma.

"Indeed," replied Randy. "How cruel of them." The rookie snickered, but no one really noticed.

"And then," she said, leaning forward, her perfect breasts curving in an exaggeration of the movement of her shoulders. "They tied me up!"

"Urggh!" grunted Randy, somehow at a loss for words.

"And then they stole my clothes!" she gasped. "All of them!" She reached out and touched the rookie's arm. He once again giggled.

"That's awful," said Randy, recovering himself. Suddenly he realized she was still naked—or rather thought she might be cold because while she told her story, her body was indicating a chill. "Jenson," he ordered, using his captain voice, "get a blanket for her, for God's sake."

Jenson ran to the engine and returned with one of the wool blankets they kept for patients in their emergency response kit. "Here, miss," said Jenson, presenting the blanket in both arms. Fortunately Johnson, who was a more seasoned firefighter, stepped forward, grasping the blanket and assisting their mermaid with her woolen shawl.

"Why, thank you, sir," she drawled, giving Johnson the look of an adoring angel.

"You'rghhhh," croaked Johnson as he turned beet red and stepped back into the lineup of maleness.

Turning back to Captain Randy, she continued her story. "And that's not all—" she said, flinging her arms wide and almost losing her newly found covering. Randy was grateful it stayed in place as he was having trouble focusing.

"Those rascals set my house on *fire!*" she said, grasping at the shawl and pulling it tight around her as a shiver shook her delicate frame.

Randy found himself refocusing at the mention of fire, but he also began to question if this wonder was quite all there upstairs. "That's awful. Did you manage to put it out?" There had been no reports of a fire anywhere that night.

"Oh no, sir." She reached out again, grasping Randy's arm this time. "And it's getting really big!"

Simmons, the engineer, leaned forward and caught his Captain's eye. He arched an eyebrow, and Randy dipped his head in agreement. Unfortunately, this unspoken dialogue in which they doubted her sanity did not escape the eye of the woman in front of them. "Why, you don't believe me!" she gasped in utter consternation.

Simmons and Captain Randy both flushed full face at being caught. "I'm sorry, ma'am." And Randy truly was. "But you have to admit that your story sounds a little...well, unusual."

"Well, I never," huffed the little angel indignantly. "All you have to do is look."

Randy now switched to his placating voice. "And where would you have us look, dear?"

Their little mermaid held his gaze firmly as she slowly extended her bare arm out from the confines of the blanket and pointed behind the line of firefighters. They all turned as one to follow her gesture, and they all froze as one upon seeing the fully involved house fire on the other side of the street, the friendly ocean breeze blowing the smoke up and away from them.

"Urck," said the Rookie.

"Shit!" yelled Simmons.

"Crap!" Johnson exclaimed.

"Get the gear, and call it in!" yelled Captain Randy.

Their naked goddess was forgotten in the recognition of their constant nemesis. Flying into action, they pulled the engine to the other side of the street, hooking to the hydrant. Additional help was responding, and someone would take care of the green-eyed naked nymph on the other side of the street while they did what they did best.

IT WAS NICE TALKING TO YOU

When she called 911, she had requested that they not send "God and everybody." That is what she told me and my partner, Joe, as she met us on the curb. "I don't want a bunch of people getting all excited for nothing."

She was the classic grandma type: graying hair that had obviously recently seen a hairstylist, a simple cotton dress, support hose, and a pair of those ugly utilitarian black shoes that elderly women seem always to wear. She held herself upright on her wooden cane, clutching a black patent-leather purse to her chest. Wobbling slightly, she was scolding her granddaughter for "trying to get involved."

"Jessica, you respect your grandmother's wishes. I told you I have called the ambulance because this is the way I want things. You are not driving me to the hospital or the doctor, and neither you nor your mother is coming with me," she chided as we stood in the sun and watched the exchange. She looked pale and tired; her knees trembled gently above the swollen ankles stuffed inside the thick support hose.

"Ma'am, you don't look like you feel very well," I said, trying to shorten the exchange before me. "Why don't we get you into the ambulance and then talk about this?"

She looked at me over the top edge of her tortoiseshell-rimmed glasses. "My dear, this is my show," she said to me, putting me gently but firmly in my place. "We will proceed at my pace." She turned back to her granddaughter and, reaching out, pulled her in for a hug. "I need you to be a good girl now and go take care of your mother." She patted her granddaughter gently on the cheek.

My partner had, in his hurry to get out of the sun, pulled the gurney from the ambulance and set it up on the sidewalk. Eyeing the bed disdainfully, my grandmotherly patient addressed Joe. "Is that really necessary?" she queried. Looking over her head at me, my partner arched his eyebrows. He was very young and had little tolerance for a slower pace.

"Yes, ma'am," I interrupted. "It is necessary. It's a safety thing." Looking back at me, she sighed and with Joe's help adjusted herself on the sheet-covered gurney. Joe adjusted the back for her sitting comfort, and together we bent to lift the gurney into loading position. "Oh my!" she exclaimed with delight, watching me lift my end of the gurney. "Look at you go," she exclaimed. "How did you get to be so strong?" I smiled at her as my partner hooked the loading rail on the gurney and lifted the legs while I held up the foot end. Pushing forward until the locking mechanisms clicked, I climbed in after her. "What a fun job you have!" she said as she reached out and patted my hand. Directing her attention out the back door of the ambulance, she again waved at her granddaughter. "Bye now, Jessica. Remember: Grandma loves you!" she hollered as Joe closed the doors

I had already pulled the blood-pressure cuff and oxygen monitor off the shelf as I addressed her. "O.K., my dear, now why did you call us?" I asked gently.

Laying her purse down across her lap, she answered thoughtfully. "Well, you see, I've been having these pains in my chest on and off for a few weeks now and feeling really not all that well, so I thought I would call you for a ride to the hospital." At the mention of chest pain, I reached out and pulled the monitor wires from the machine. Unbuttoning the front of her dress, I applied the three electrodes as we spoke.

"Why didn't you call the doctor sooner?" I asked as I looked at her cardiac rhythm march out across the little screen. It was showing a depressed segment that would indicate a possibility that the chest pain she had been experiencing was a heart attack.

We had about a ten-minute drive to the hospital from this location, and my hands moved to set up an IV as I sought more information. Reaching out, she grasped my hands and held them gently. "Let's not get all excited now, shall we? It doesn't hurt right now." She smiled up at me. "I need to show you some papers first." Letting go of my hands, she reached into her shiny black purse and pulled out a bundle of papers that she spread out over the top of her bag. "I went to my lawyer this morning, and he assures me this is all very legal," she explained in her grandmotherly voice. "This part here says that I do not want any heroic methods taken to prolong my life. That includes IVs, medications, electricity, ventilators—" Picking up the paperwork, she read the rest. "'—intubation, or compressions.' We are going to let God have his way."

Reaching out, I took the papers and examined them closely. It was a legal do-not-resuscitate order signed by my patient on that day's date. "Wow," I said, slightly taken aback. "Why? You seem healthy enough."

Smiling at me gently, she spoke slowly and quietly, obviously wanting me to understand. "You see," she explained, "my Daniel passed away six months ago. He was the love of my life. No, no, he *was* my life. We had been married over sixty years, and until that night we never slept apart." She continued on, telling me of their life together—the joys and sorrows they had shared in a life that was full and complete. She spoke of the town we were in and all the changes they had seen there. They had watched it grow as they raised their family together.

I interrupted only once to ask if her daughter and granddaughter wouldn't miss her. "Why, of course," she replied, once again making me feel as if I were confused.

I quickly called in my report to the hospital, including the details of the DNR orders, and she then continued her story. She had a calming voice, and I listened intently as she described her life.

Her story nearing completion with the death of her beloved Daniel, she reached out her hand and placed it gently on my knee. Laying her head back on the pillow, she sighed. "Sweetie," she said, patting my knee gently, "it's been wonderful talking to you, but I'm afraid I have to go now." She closed her eyes and sighed again.

Confused, I pulled back and looked at her. What an odd thing to say! And then I realized she had stopped breathing. Adrenaline kicked hard at me as my eyes flew to my monitor. My wonderful companion's heart was in ventricular fibrillation. Unless I used electricity to stop the erratic rhythm, she would be dead in just a few minutes! And as I reached for the paddles of my monitor to apply the needed shock, her paperwork, which I had laid on the bench seat next to me, fell to the floor.

I froze in my actions. Bending, I picked up the papers and examined them again. Looking up at her gentle, peaceful face, I realized that she had known. She had known all along.

She had seen her lawyer that morning. She wouldn't let the family come with her. This was, as she had said, her show, and it was well choreographed.

Holding the cluster of papers on my lap, I leaned back against the bench seat as the backup alarm started to sound. We were at the hospital.

"I'M NOT PREGNANT!"

I t was 6:00 a.m. Shift change was scheduled for an hour later. My partner and I were exhausted. We had been up all night running calls, most of them for people who had developed a case of the stomach flu that was working its way through the city. It had always amazed me what people would call an ambulance for: an ankle that had been sprained over a week ago, a backache, cold symptoms for a week, or the stomach flu. I had been raised to believe that ambulances were for life-threatening emergencies only and had never gotten used to the idea that some people found nasal congestion to be a true emergency. Part of the problem was the mistaken belief that if you went to the hospital by ambulance, you wouldn't have to wait so long. Initially that may have been true, but the hospitals had figured out a long time ago that people were abusing the system to avoid the wait. Now people who misused ambulances usually ended up waiting even longer than the people who drove themselves to the hospital for non-emergencies. The EDs referred to this as a "therapeutic wait," and it was an effort to curb the abuse of the system. Still the fallacy persisted, and people would tell us they had called only to avoid the lobby. In California, the law required ambulances to take anyone to the hospital who requested it. It caused problems. For the last twenty-four hours, we had been driving people to the hospital who had the stomach flu and were vomiting and suffering from diarrhea—sometimes with symptoms for less than an hour. The system was stretched to the limit, and we were exhausted.

The tones had announced the same symptoms that we had been transporting all that day and the day before. "Medic engine ten, medic 132, respond to a nineteen-year-old female with nausea and stomach pain."

The fire station was located just around the corner from the address given on the call, and the engine beat us there by two to three minutes. As we were pulling up, the captain from the engine met us at the ambulance. "I really hope this stomach flu passes soon. The guys are walking her down. She's a big one." He sounded as tired as we felt.

Looking up the stairwell of the apartment building, we were greeted by the site of a huge woman making her way down the steps. She must have weighed close to three hundred pounds, and the firefighters were hidden behind her bulk as she descended the stairs.

"Oh my God!" moaned by partner from behind me. "My back hurts already."

The fire captain who had greeted us chuckled as we pulled the gurney around and had the large woman sit on the bed. The lifting was fairly easy with four people, with one of us on each corner. The fire-department paramedic had gathered the important information from the patient as they had walked her down the stairs, and he now relayed it to me. "She's nineteen years old and has been nauseated for a few days. She says she has been constipated for several weeks. She also says her stomach hurts. We haven't taken any vital signs yet. She was waiting for us at the door."

"Well," I thought, "at least it's not the stomach flu again if she's constipated."

Climbing into the back of the ambulance, I surveyed my patient. I had offered to ride with her on the way over. Both my partner and I wanted to get back to the station and go home. I had the most experience and figured I could whip out the paperwork on the way to the hospital, allowing us the extra few minutes to hopefully get off shift on time.

The firefighter closed the door and waved good-bye as I pulled out the biggest blood-pressure cuff and did a quick check on my patient. She wasn't a very friendly sort, and after confirming the information that the fire medic had given me, I sat back to do my paperwork. I blamed the nagging feeling that something was not right on my exhausted state.

One of the most important lessons that a new paramedic learns is to listen to the sixth sense, that little voice in your head that tells you to pay closer attention. My little voice was yelling at me, and glancing at the patient, I wondered again why. I thought to myself that maybe my little voice just hadn't had enough sleep either. I went back to my paperwork but just couldn't focus. The persistent little voice was not letting me concentrate. I laid the tag book aside and addressed my patient. Obviously, I was missing something.

"So tell me again what's going on?"

The young woman stared out the back doors of the ambulance. "I told you," she said. "I've got the constipation, and I don't feel good."

"O.K., my dear, tell you what," I said, trying to keep this light. The patient was obviously in no mood for conversation. "I need to feel your stomach and make sure I'm not missing anything. O.K.?" Without looking at me she nodded affirmation. I placed my hands on the patient's large stomach and felt the different landmarks. It was hard to tell through all the rolls of fat, but nothing seemed unusual. Her stomach was soft—nothing unusual except for one small area that felt tight. But if she was constipated, that too would be normal. I thought to myself that I was too tired as I picked my tag book back up and returned to the paperwork.

Still the little voice would not leave me alone. "This is ridiculous!" I thought, getting angry with myself. "All right, we do *all* the questions." Again, I laid my tag book to the side.

"Dear, I know you don't feel well, but I need to ask you a few more questions." My patient still didn't look at me, so I continued. "Have you ever had a stomachache like this before?" No answer. "When was the last time you saw your doctor?"

This time she answered, "Last week. He said I've got the constipation and gas problems."

Fatigue made me want to giggle, but I suppressed it and continued. "What type of gas problems did he say you have?"

My patient's eyes stayed focused on the road behind us. "He said I've got bloating."

The fatigue was fighting against the serious voice, but the voice won out. I continued with the text book questions. "Did he find anything else wrong with you?"

"No," she replied.

I asked about medications that he might have given her. Nothing. "Have you ever been pregnant or had female problems?" I asked.

This time, for the first time during our ride, my patient made eye contact with me. "I ain't got no kids, and I'm not pregnant." Too fast and too strong.

Picking up the tag book to diffuse her anxiety about the questions, I continued. "These questions are for the doctor. He is going to ask me what is wrong, and I need to be able to tell him. When was your last period?"

My patient was again looking out the back of the ambulance. "I started this morning," she said.

I was lost. I knew better than to ignore my little voice, but I just wasn't getting anywhere. Again I reached out and palpated her large belly. "And are your periods normal?"

She paused before she answered. "No, they ain't been normal for a long time, but they been there."

"O.K., maybe now we are getting somewhere," I thought and then continued with my questions. "How long since they've been normal, dear?"

She made eye contact again. "They ain't been normal since August." My brain was awake now as I counted off the months in my head: August, September, October, November, December, January, February, March, April. Nine Months!

Reaching out to touch the patient's hand, I gently asked the big question. "Dear, could you be pregnant?"

My patient yanked her hand out from under mine. The anger was in her eyes as she answered my question. "I ain't pregnant! I told you; I need to have a bowel movement. I'm constipated."

She was angry, but I had to finish the question. "Is there *any* chance you could be pregnant?" I asked.

"You don' listen, does you?" my patient responded. "I ain't pregnant. There ain't no chance I is pregnant. I ain't had sex with no one in a long time."

My large patient obviously needed a few minutes to calm down, and I needed to tell the hospital what I was thinking. I moved to the front of the ambulance and reached for the microphone to the hospital. "I've already called it in," my partner said.

"Yeah, I know." I also knew how this was going to sound. "But I've changed my mind about what is wrong." My partner turned down the FM radio to listen in. This was going to sound so stupid, but it had to be done. My little voice hadn't let me down in ten years; it couldn't be wrong this time. "County base, this is Medic twelve. Update on our nineteen-year-old female..." I paused. They were not going to believe me, and I knew it. "County, this is going to sound stupid, but I think this patient is in labor."

The radio crackled back at me. "Medic twelve, patient's due date, and how far apart are the contractions?"

I thought to myself that I had better be right as I continued. "Uh, county, patient denies any possibility of being pregnant, and I can't feel any contractions." There was a long pause on the radio. I knew what they were thinking. I knew how stupid that sounded, but if I was right, they needed some warning.

"Ten four, medic twelve. We'll just see you when you get here."

My partner grinned in the rearview mirror at me and chuckled. "That sounded professional," he said. Well, I didn't blame them. Part of me didn't believe me either. Now my stomach was starting to hurt. "Maybe I just need a long vacation," I thought as I moved back to my patient's side.

I was rechecking my patient's blood pressure and feeling a little sorry for myself when she started to wiggle around on the gurney. "I've got to go to the bathroom now!" There was a touch of desperation in her voice as she spoke. I watched her strain the sides of the gurney with her gyrations.

"Well," I thought, "it's all or nothing." Grabbing the sides of her stretch pants, I pulled down. "I have to check something, dear. Lift your bottom." With her help I managed to drag her pants down around her knees. Standing up, I pushed the rolls of fat out of the way as I checked my patient. She was bulging at the perineum, and a small trickle of fluid escaped her vagina. I caught the musky smell of childbirth and knew I was right. "Sweetie, whatever you do, don't push."

"But I've got to go to the bathroom bad," she said as she strained and pulled on the arms of the gurney.

"*No!*" I said. "Whatever you do, *don't push!*"

The beeping sound of the backup alarm heralded our arrival at the hospital as I tore open an OB kit. I pulled the sterile gloves from the kit and snapped them into place. My patient was now holding her legs wide open and bearing down. The head of the baby showed as the battle of childbirth continued. "Stop pushing!" I ordered as my partner opened the doors in the back. I threw the OB kit on the back of the gurney.

Quickly appraising the situation, my partner asked, "Here or inside?"

"Inside," I told him. "We don't know for sure that it's term, and she's had no prenatal care. We may need help."

Quickly we pulled the gurney from the ambulance and headed into the emergency department. My assumption that they wouldn't believe my crazy report was right, but the smile on the face of the receiving nurse disappeared as we rushed in. "She crowning!" I said. They were not expecting this. "She still says she is not pregnant," I said.

The ED doctor had been listening to the whole exchange and sprang quickly into action. Assessing my patient, he ordered the nurses to call the OB department. "Let them know we're coming up. Unknown due date." One of the ER nurses ran beside us as we headed for the elevators.

My patient began to push from side to side, almost tipping the gurney. Glancing down, I saw the head of the baby slip from its confines into the world. "Stop!" I yelled.

The doctor who was leading the parade turned. Reaching out, he took the baby's head into his hands. "Suction," he said. I pulled the small bulb syringe from the back of the gurney and suctioned the new infant's nose and mouth.

My patient grimaced again. "*I am not pregnant!*" The echo of her voice bounced off the walls of the corridors.

The doctor's voice was firm as he responded. "Give it a minute, and you won't be."

The baby boy made his entrance into the world there in the hospital corridor. The mother stared at the wall of the hospital as we clamped and clipped the umbilical cord. I carried the wiggling little boy as our entourage, plus one, continued up the elevator to the OB floor. They were ready for us and herded us into a delivery room. Handing the baby to one of the nurses, I helped my partner move our patient over to the hospital bed. The nurse who had taken the baby checked him over quickly and pronounced that he appeared to be full term. She moved back to the side of the hospital bed next to the mother.

"Don't you want to see your son?" I asked.

My patient's eyes were filled with anger as she looked accusingly first at me and then the doctor. Slowly her angry eyes fell on her newborn son. Not a sound emanated from the room as we all held our breaths.

The anger faded. Tears formed in the corners of her eyes as a smile began to form on her lips. Her hand trembled just slightly as she reached tentatively out and brushed the head of her newborn son for the first time.

She may not have wanted to be pregnant, but the look on her face relieved my fears. These two would be just fine.

SICK DAY

I woke up this morning with a sore throat, headache, tight chest, and general aches and pains. I am sure I have a fever. I don't have to check it, and I don't want to check it (just in case it's ninety-eight point six) because I feel sick. That is enough for me. I am going to stay in bed like God intended and read books, sleep, drink orange juice, and maybe even watch some stupid TV reruns from thirty years ago. I like to think that God invented colds to allow us to stay in bed for the day.

I am not going to call the doctor or an ambulance for a ride to the emergency department because I don't feel good. I have never understood why anyone would even want to do that. I am always curious whether those in our society who do this have never been sick before. Have they never experienced the comforts of lying in bed under the weight of piles of comforters, not answering the phone, and just letting nature take its course? Sometimes I wonder if it is possible that all of the people that come to the ER when they have a cold or flu were deprived in childhood. Maybe they have never known the comfort of Mom kissing their forehead to check for a fever or the smell of homemade chicken noodle soup simmering in the kitchen. Maybe that is why they come to us when they should be home under all those blankets, experiencing the luxury of feeling sorry for themselves and knowing that they are blessed with a simple cold.

At the ER we give them warm blankets and *oh* and *ah* over their symptoms. We give them fluid to drink and check their temperature (although not with a kiss to the forehead). However, they also run the risk of getting a grumpy nurse or a doc who has the same cold and did not stay home. This could include the raised eyebrows that greet the woeful description of their phlegm as the care provider nonverbally compares the severity of the patient's illness with his or her own agony. The caregiver should have stayed home too. There is no joy in the comparison of discomfort.

One of the joys of childhood was Mom believing the exaggeration of the cold symptoms and allowing us to stay home and hibernate. It meant no math class and an excuse to make up that spelling test we hadn't studied for anyway. So why, as adults, do we deviate from the gift of that? We don't even have to exaggerate the symptoms; we only have to believe that there is no human on the face of the earth that is too important to reschedule a meeting or have someone else cover a shift. There are few gifts as comfortably paedomorphic as staying in bed all day under a pile of quilts in a fetal position.

"WE JUST WANT TO SAY GOOD-BYE"

The family had brought her into the hospital the night before she had been transferred to ICU. She had been having severe abdominal pain, and the family was worried. She weighed not more than eighty pounds, and her delicate skin pulled tight around her skeleton. She was the matriarch of the family. They called her Momma.

Momma had spent most of the night undergoing diagnostic tests. Her abdominal pain had been diagnosed as cholecystitis, or in layman's terms, gallbladder problems. Momma had been admitted to surgery immediately, but the gallbladder had been found to be so necrosed that she had been sewn back up still intact.

Momma had lived a good life. She was eighty-nine years old and had survived both a heart attack and several strokes over the years. Her family had refused to send her to a convalescent hospital and instead kept her at home and shared her care. Momma couldn't speak anymore, and the family told the nurses that the moans and an occasional scream were her way of communicating. Before they left the hospital, the family had signed the DNR papers, orders to not take heroic measures should Momma pass away. They were friendly with the nurses on staff and had pleaded with them to call immediately if it looked as if Momma was going to "cross over so that they could say good-bye."

Shelly was assigned to Momma and wasn't surprised when at approximately ten o'clock that evening, the alarms sounded in the room. Rushing in, Shelly found that not only was Momma not breathing with any regularity, but she also had weak pulses, which corresponded to an abnormally slow rhythm on the cardiac monitor. Momma was dying.

Remembering her promise to Momma's family, Shelly called for assistance from one of the other nurses and rushed to the phone to call the family.

"Oh, please, don't let her die until we get there," the family begged. "We want to be with her and say good-bye."

How could Shelly refuse? The family obviously loved this frail little woman dearly. Life was her dedication, and saying good-bye to it in the right way made things easier on everyone. "Of course, but please hurry."

Shelly returned to the room where Momma lay. Momma had stopped breathing on her own, and the nurse who was with her was helping the failing matriarch breathe with a bag-valve mask. Shelly's heart sunk. "Oh man, Gloria. I'm sorry, but I just promised the family that we would keep her alive until they get here. Can you stay and help?" Gloria agreed, and together they used the bag-valve device to breathe for Momma. Her heart rate was still slow, but with the continual assistance breathing, it kept its slow, steady pace. Five minutes turned into ten and then fifteen. Shelly and Gloria were both exhausted by the time the family showed up. All fifteen members of the family walked into Momma's room with tears in their eyes and sadness straining their faces.

"Thank you, ma'am." A man around fifty, possibly Momma's son, spoke for the family. "Thank you so much. It's so important for us to be together at this time."

The weariness left the arms of the nurses with that statement. "Anything to help your family get through this difficult time," Shelly assured the man.

The family gathered in a tight circle around Momma's bed, some holding hands and a few just crying softly. Gloria and Shelly watched as Momma's heart rate slowed to the point where there was only a flat line showing on the monitor. Shelly felt for a pulse to confirm what she knew. "Gloria, would you go notify the doctor, please?" Shelly gave her fellow nurse the exit cue. "We're going to give you all some privacy," she explained to the family as she pulled the curtain closed.

Gloria had just hung up the phone after notifying the doctor of the death. "Doc says he'll sign in the morning. Hey, Shelly, with the family in there watching the monitors, maybe we should sit her up a little bit. That way she won't have any agonal beats. We don't want to make this any more difficult than it has to be on that family."

The physiological reason was a mystery to the nurses, but it seemed to be true that sitting a recently deceased person in a semisitting position stopped the heart from having extra beats after death. These beats are normal but can be quite distracting to an untrained person watching a monitor over a bed.

"Good idea, Gloria." Shelly felt silly that she hadn't thought of it herself as she walked back into the room. "Excuse me," she said, addressing the family, "I don't mean to bother, but I thought it might be easier for you to see her face if we raised the bed a little." Shelly had learned from years of experience that it sometimes didn't hurt to candy coat the truth a little, especially for a family in mourning.

Shelly took the control panel in her hand and raised the bed slightly. Some of the family watched; most had their eyes turned down.

"Yeeeawwwwww!" It was Momma. She had thrown herself upright in the bed, opened her eyes, and began screaming. "Yeeeaaawww," went Momma.

"Yeeeaaawwwww," went the whole family in chorus.

"Oh my God!" screamed Shelly.

Gloria ran in through the doorway. "What the—"

She watched as the monitor went from flat line to a slow, normal rhythm. Rushing to the bed, she helped Momma lay back against the cushions. The family had all pulled to the back of the room with their mouths hanging open and their eyes stretched wide.

Momma lay back in silence, and her weak eyes shut. The monitor showed a regular yet slow beat of the heart, and Shelly felt a pulse in the woman's arm. Her color, though still pale, pinked up as she started breathing on her own.

The family was finally calmed down with sympathy and cool drinks. They left the hospital fatigued but gratified to the two angels in white, again obtaining promises that they would be called should Momma show signs of leaving her earthly existence.

The doctor was called. The situation was explained to him, and Momma spent the next twenty-four hours with no changes. She had indeed shown improvement for the first twelve hours, with an increased pulse rate and higher oxygen levels.

As the morning again dawned in the ICU, Momma began to fade. First the pulse slowed, than the breathing stopped. The family was called again by an apologetic staff who helped to maintain Momma's breathing until the grief-stricken family arrived. Again, they all gathered around the bed and mourned Momma's passing. And again, Momma's eyes popped open, and she began to moan. The family moaned in chorus as they backed away from the bed. Horrified, the family watched as the nurses again tucked Momma in and excused themselves to the nurses' station with apologies and explanations that didn't really matter at that point.

The next evening, Momma again began to deteriorate. Her breathing had slowed to an agonizing rate, and the cardiac monitor showed that her heart was weakening to the point where she would not be around much longer. The ever-vigilant and caring nurses again called the family with the bad news. They worked with Momma until the family arrived. Once again, all fifteen family members gathered around the solemn bedside. Once again, the family held back their tears and waited for the inevitable.

And…Momma got better. Slowly her heart rate increased to an acceptable level. She was breathing deeply again, raising her oxygen levels and pinking her gray complexion. The family waited around Momma's bed for an hour. Momma just kept getting better.

Once again the family praised the nurses for their caring nature and returned home. Once again the family elicited promises that they would be called should Momma near death. Once again the family left the hospital to go home and wait.

The next morning, the alarms in Momma's room sounded their insistent cry. Shelly silenced the alarms from the desk. She watched through the glass enclosure. Calling the doctor on the phone, he said what she was thinking. "Make sure this time." And Shelly watched. By eight o'clock, the monitor showed a flat line and no breathing from Momma. Shelly waited ten minutes to feel for a pulse. There was no pulse, but this was Momma. Shelly waited until eight thirty to call the family, who promised they would be right over.

Two and a half hours later, the family showed up. Not all fifteen this time, just a few.

Shelly asked if they wanted to go in and say good-bye to Momma.

The elderly man who had become the spokesperson the first night glanced into the windowed room where Momma lay. His eyes were wide as he spoke. "No," he said, shaking his gray head, "I think maybe we had better just sign the papers and let Momma rest."

WOULD YOU LIKE SOME JUICE?

It was another crazy Friday night downtown. I was working the ED, and we were slammed as usual. Gurneys lined the hallways, the triage lobby was full, ambulances were lined up outside, and all of this was taking place to a cacophony of screams and moans emanating from the various rooms. There was also a full moon coming up soon, which meant it wouldn't end until morning. So we kept plugging away, doing what we could for some and trying to reassure the rest that we would get to them as soon as possible. Sometimes it was difficult trying to explain the art of triage and treatment to people who wanted their turn in the order they had arrived. We didn't work on a take-a-number system here.

Eddie had come in by ambulance. He was a large man, over six foot four and at least four hundred pounds. His feet hung over the end of the gurney as he waited. The report said his family had called because he was acting strangely—no specifics, just strangely. In an ED this busy, that meant he had his blood-sugar levels checked along with his basic vitals, and then if all was within normal limits, he had to sit and wait with everyone else while the heart attacks, stabbings, gunshot wounds, and accident victims were treated. So Eddie sat quietly on the hallway gurney, waiting and waiting.

I had just come back from X-ray with another patient when I heard yelling at the other end of the hallway. Maneuvering around the people left waiting in the hallway who were straining to see what was happening, I rushed to help. Eddie had climbed over the railing on the side of the gurney and was jumping up and down in the hallway. In between jumps, he was pulling his clothes off. His pants were lying crumpled on the floor; his shirt went flying and caught on the IV pole at the head of the gurney. His shoes and socks were long gone. And then his shorts were too! Yes, there was Eddie in all of his naked glory in the middle of the hallway. The only people who moved were the caregivers, nurses, and techs. But Eddie was having none of it. Screaming at the top of his lungs, he punched one of the approaching nurses in the face, sending her flying. An aide tripped over a second patient as Eddie shoved her sideways down the hall.

Eddie bellowed again and, like an angry bull, charged for the ambulance-bay doors. The hallway cleared before him as patients and nurses scrambled out of his way. The doors slid open, and naked Eddie rushed out into the night air with one of the male nurses and a doctor in close pursuit. I ran after them into the darkness and down a side street that was lined on one side by the hospital and on the other by the local cemetery.

The street was dark, and the only part of Eddie that could be seen with clarity was his pumping buttocks as he ran down the center of the street. Ron, the nurse, was obviously in better shape than Eddie and caught up with him about a hundred feet down the road. But Eddie was having none of it. As Ron's hand reached out to restrain him, Eddie's fist came up yet again, sending Ron flying onto the sidewalk. Dr. Everett approached next, speaking to Eddie in a gentle voice, but Eddie would have none of it. His bellows echoed off the walls of the hospital and down the street as he charged the doctor, sending him onto his back also. Eddie's enraged face came up, and he saw me standing about twenty feet away. Too late, I realized the error of my way as the bull-charge bellow again rose in Eddie's throat. His naked feet slapped the pavement as he lowered his head and charged toward me.

I wish I could say that I reasoned it out or that my training took over and I subdued the beast with my superior people skills, but the truth is that I simply stood still in the path of destruction and said the first thing that came to my mind. "Eddie, would you like some juice?"

Eddie slammed to a halt just feet from me. He froze in all his naked glory, his male parts bobbing in the dark. "What?" he said.

I am not a small woman, but Eddie dwarfed me as he stood looking down at me. Standing stock still, I tilted my head back and looked up into his stunned face. "I said, would you like some juice? We have several kinds."

In my mind the moment took forever as Eddie studied me slowly. I was half the size of the doctor he had just sent sprawling and no challenge to him as I stood there in my cute decorative scrubs. "Yeah," Eddie said at last, "Yeah, that would be good."

"We have cranberry, orange, and apple," I said, like a waitress on a weird planet of naked monsters.

"Can I have one of each?" Eddie asked in a quiet little voice that sounded like a small boy.

"Sure, Eddie. But it's inside. We have to go back in," I said. Where was the security guard when you needed them?

"O.K.," said Eddie. "Will you hold my hand?" he asked, extending his baseball-mitt-sized hand toward me.

"Sure, Eddie," I said, reaching out and slipping my hand into the giant grip of the naked behemoth. Eddie's giant mitt closed over my hand as we turned to walk back up the street toward the ED. The moon had just started to come up over the silhouette of the tombstones in the adjoining graveyard, casting weird shadows as I walked beside this naked hulk. He held my hand in his, my head not even coming to his shoulder as we plodded past the doctor and the nurse, and past the gaping security guards into the ambulance-bay doors of the ED.

The busy ED again went quiet as I walked in beside my now-mellow, naked giant. I led him to a waiting gurney and provided Eddie with not only one of each juice but also a sandwich and some chips.

He sat quietly in the hall and consumed his fare. The triage order was changed to accommodate his staunch refusal to put his clothing back on, and after an accelerated evaluation, Eddie was given a nice, safe, naked ambulance ride to the psychiatric facility down the street.

FAMILY

S he was not that old. Fairly young really, although *young* can be a relative term in the art of medicine. She had a cardiac bypass and was doing fine...for a while. Then she seemed to fade. It happens sometimes. People have underlying medical problems that are exacerbated by invasive therapy. That was a nice way to say that the operation was too hard on her and that she didn't have the resources to survive such an extensive surgery.

She must have been a great mother. Her family was all at the bedside. Some of them had flown in from parts far away to be with their mom.

The other nurses said that for several days after the surgery, she had been doing great—joking around and laughing with her family. The first day I had her, she was back on a ventilator, which provided the breaths that her body required to stay alive. However, her body (or God) had decided she'd had enough. Her lungs rattled with accumulated fluids and infection as I listened to them. Her legs, where the incisions had been, oozed with reddish-tinged fluids. Her laughter was silenced when the doctors replaced the tube to keep her airway open and placed her on a ventilator because her body was too sick to keep breathing on its own.

I spent the day doing routine ICU care. I swabbed her mouth, suctioned the tube that kept her trachea receptive to breaths, and adjusted her IVs and all the drugs that dripped through them to keep her tired heart pumping. Then her son wanted to know if I would talk to him. Of course, it's just part of the job. He asked me if I thought she was getting better. "No," I replied, "she is staying the same, according to the reports I have received. She is a very sick lady."

He was a grown man in a tailored business suit, yet his leg swung out, and his head bowed in a posture of a frightened child as he asked me if she would get better. Oh God. I had never lied to a patient or family. Yet not wanting to allow myself to feel the pain of what he was going to feel, I answered ambiguously, "From the reports that I received, she seem to be holding her own for now." That wasn't good enough. Days of denial and politically correct sidestepping by the staff had made him persistent.

He moved a step closer. "How's Mom really doing? Why won't anyone tell me the truth?"

Sepsis and disseminated intravascular coagulation was how she was doing. Terms he wouldn't understand. She was dying because her body was slowly shutting down due to an infection somewhere inside. How do you explain to a dying woman's son something that took you at least a semester of college to understand?

Again I tried to take the easy route. "The doctor will be here soon. If you have concerns, you should speak with him."

Not to be outdone, he countered my parry. "We have been trying to reach the doctor for four days. He does not return our calls, and he never comes in when we are here with Mom."

He had trumped my ace. "Has the doctor talked to you at all?"

He looked down and replied in a very quiet voice, "Not since four days ago!"

I was a nurse. More than a nurse, I was a person who had a family of my own. I recognized the primal fear of loss and of the exquisite pain that accompanies the reality of death when I saw it. This man was hurting, which made him my patient too.

I gathered his extended hand in mine and told him, "She is very lucky to have you here. You need to stay with her. She is very tired, and you need to know that."

He seemed to understand as the tears welled up in his eyes. We all live in denial to a degree. I am not sure we could face the daily chore of continued existence if we didn't.

I gave him the introduction, and somewhere deep inside, he knew the script.

"Thank you," he said. "Thank you. I will go get the others." He started to walk away, and then turned and, with eyes brimming, asked, "Will you let us in? The night nurses said we were disturbing Mom's rest."

The rules were strict, but death did not need privacy to happen, and I assured him that as long as I was on shift, his family would be with his mother.

She stayed the night. I went home to indulge myself in the quiet and need of my family, so bittersweet when I watched life and death unfold daily.

At 7:00 a.m., I received report from the night nurse. "The family is just impossible!" she said. "I couldn't get anything done. They kept holding her hands and standing in the way. I finally had to make them go to the lobby."

She was very young, and I knew she would not understand if I tried to explain. I received the numbers and lab reports from her as fast as I could and then excused myself from the desk. My shift began at 7:00 a.m., but the ICU was closed until eight to offer privacy for reports and doctors' visits without interruption. Sometimes the rules ceased to matter. I walked straight to the ICU waiting room. The son was not there, but the eyes of my patient's daughter widened with fear when she saw me walk toward her. I held out my hands in the universal sign of denial. "Your mom is still here, but she needs you. I came to get you. You need to be with her now."

"She's not going to make it, is she?"

Oh, my heart broke at moments like this. I was not God and had no idea what he was going to determine. My professional experience said that no, she was not going to stay here. However, what if I said that, and God—or whatever power that was—determined otherwise?

"I don't know that, but my heart tells me that if she were my mom, I would want to be there with her. Please come back. I am her nurse for today, and I will tell everyone that it is O.K."

She grabbed my hands in hers, and her blue eyes locked mine. "But you're breaking rules for us. Why?"

"Because she needs you there...because you love her...that's all."

"So why did the night nurse—?"

I cut her off there. I had my own beliefs of life and death, but I wouldn't allow myself to disparage the new nurses. The ones that didn't know yet, that hadn't seen. They would learn and grow. We all did.

"It doesn't matter now. I'm here until tonight, and I believe your Mother would want you there. Since I am her nurse, it is a done deal."

She followed me into the recesses of the ICU, with its beeping alarms and swooshing beat of ventilators prolonging the inevitable. She held her mother and sang songs with her sister around the bedside until her mother was no more. Her brother had joined her by then, and his tenor added to the quiet hymns they sang for a safe passage. They cried and loved with a passion that only occurs at the presence of death and the realization of loss. I allowed the tears to creep down my cheeks with their pain. It was not willingly—I always tried not to cry—but sometimes the power of the pain felt by those who love overwhelmed even those of us who should have been callous enough to withstand it. When it became too much, I stepped out of the room to "check the labs" or to "check on my other patient," although the other ICU nurses automatically assumed the care of other patients at a time like this. It gave me time to assure myself that I could be strong for those in need. For those who were losing someone they loved.

Her family surrounded her as she took her last breaths. I had turned off the monitors in the room to allow a peaceful, quiet moment. Life does not end suddenly for most but only in steps. As her body assumed the dusky hue that precedes death, she held the hands of those she loved. She was ushered into the realm that awaits us with the sounds of her favorite hymns sung by the voices of those she had brought into the world.

There are good deaths, and there are bad deaths. Healthcare providers are the ushers that assist the families through the darkened aisles of the theater in which death performs. We hide in the shadows of the stage, awaiting the curtain call that signals the end, and most often we cry with joy for a life well lived, with disappointment in a passing, with shared sadness.

CAT WOMAN

" **S**o I need you to go out and talk to her. The county goes out there a lot; public health about once a year. She has a son and a daughter who call every time they come to town. She hasn't let anyone in that house in ten years—including her family—so we don't expect much, but her daughter knows people who know people, and they want us to check on the sores on her legs. It's a request from the adult protective division of the DAs office. Just talk to her, look at her legs, and file a report." Since I was the new guy, my boss often handed me the assignments she found less than desirable. Fortunately, her idea of onerous duty and mine differed greatly, although I was in no way going to let her know that. In fact, I was happy to comply. Working public health had its benefits due to the diversity of the departmental responsibilities, but it could still get a little redundant at times, and this offered a nice, if short, change of pace.

Taking the keys for one of the generic county cars, I grabbed my medical bag, my purse, and the paperwork I would need. Last stop was for the cheap county-issue cell phone, which I put in the pocket of my lab coat and headed out the door. It was good to be outside again. After so many years of working as a medic, I often found the confines of hospital and office to be a bit overwhelming. I tossed my stuff in the passenger seat, rolled down the windows, and checked my map. I was a little disappointed to find that the location was in town as I loved driving out into the country on days like this. I made a quick stop at the local 7-11 store for a bottle of water and drove to the house. Arriving fifteen minutes before the scheduled meeting time with the representative from adult protective, I settled back in my seat and had a look at this mystery house that no one had been in for ten years. Basically it was one of those wonderful old farmhouses with arching windows and a wraparound porch that had survived the ranch-style house invasion of the '60s and '70s. Looking a bit run down with peeling white paint and windows dimmed by dust, it sat in the middle of a huge lot. Two old oaks grew in the extended front yard. A white iron garden bench was tucked cozily between the two and in the midst of a bed of out-of-control irises. Three or four cats sunned themselves on the porch, and two kittens played among the overgrown irises.

The scene was relaxing, and I let my mind wander into a fantasy of the inside of such a house. The attention to detail of the architects who designed houses in centuries past fascinated me, and I loved indulging in the guessing game of what unique treasures had been placed into such houses. The arriving social worker chuckled when I jumped at her welcome next to my open window.

"Sorry," I said as I popped the door and climbed out of the car. "I was off in my own little world."

"It's a good day for it," she said as she introduced herself. "Just so you know, we won't get in."

We stood in the sun by my county car as she explained the history. "Her kids have been calling once or twice a year for the last ten years. This past year, it has accelerated. Every month now. We take turns coming out. I've been out here myself three times now, and Mrs. Colt is quite honestly a nut. Half the time, she doesn't even open the door, just yells at us through the window. She's been living here by herself since her husband died twelve years ago. Her daughter was in the house about ten years ago and called us about trying to make her mom get rid of her cats." She pointed to the ones lazing in the sun on the porch. "She must have hundreds of them in there," she said, indicating the house. "Her daughter called again last week complaining that she was out here to visit, and her mom has sores all over her legs. Mom wouldn't let her in the door. I'm not sure what exactly she thinks we can do about it, but it takes the responsibility off of her to send us out again. The woman pays her bills and her taxes and hasn't bothered anyone yet. Technically the house is over the city line, so there are no restrictions on the number of cats she can own." She leaned back against my car as a sheriff patrol unit pulled in behind us. "I thought maybe a little law-enforcement appearance might help us get a look," she said as the officer got out of his car and approached.

Just then the door to the house opened, and a small woman flowed out of the house in a wave of cats with a little red wagon in tow. She bent and shooed two of the cats back in, leaving the rest to do as they pleased. She was wearing an old blue housedress with a faded floral print that extended below her knees and mismatched bobby socks with flat tennis shoes that had probably been white at one time. Even from this distance I could see the red areas of her legs rising above her socks and peeking out from under the faded housedress. Her eyes squinted as she looked out in our direction at the gathering of cars and strangers. The relaxed, at-home manner changed abruptly as her eyes focused on the invaders of her domain. She disappeared back into the house with a bang of the door, leaving the cats and the little red wagon sitting on the porch.

"Hummm," rumbled the officer. "I told the sergeant I don't know why you called us out here again. She ain't hurtin' no one, and she ain't broke no laws."

I held my tongue as the DA representative and the officer began to argue back and forth about the merits of "bringin' the law down" on little old ladies. Curtain shadows indicated observation by cats, Mrs. Colt, or both as the discussion went nowhere.

"Excuse me," I interrupted. "Why don't I go see if she will at least let me take a look at her legs? I'm pretty good with people. Let's try simple first." The officer leaned back against my car as he happily accepted my solution. DA lady however insisted that she had to talk to Mrs. Colt so she too could file a report.

Leaving the officer to sun himself against the side of my car, we walked up the weed-filled drive to the porch. The neglect of lawn and house loomed larger as we approached. The collage of cats skittered off around the side and under the porch at the approach of strangers, yet the odor of them lingered there. The sharp, musky smell of cat urine defeated the summer breeze that offered to push it off the porch, and we were left standing at the door in a perfume of eau de cat. Pushing the doorbell produced no sound, and we resorted to knocking. "Emma. Open the door," my companion ordered.

The curtains that had fallen into place as we approached again ruffled to the side of the window. "Go away!" Her voice was soft but firm. No flowery excuses. Just her wishes.

"Now, Emma, you know I can't do that until we talk." My companion used a tone of voice that reminded me of an unloved school teacher. "Your daughter called again, and we have to check on you."

"You ain't getting in! I recognize you. You been here afore. You got no business. Leave me be, and tell my daughter to mind her own beeswax." I smiled inside at the ferociousness in her old voice as she left no option open.

"Now, Mrs.—"

I stopped my companion with a hand on her arm. "Let me try, please. Mrs. Colt, I have not been here before," I started. "I'm a registered nurse, and my only concern is those sores on your legs."

Silence followed my statement. "Mrs. Colt?" I said.

The door eased open with a chain securely in place, and one eye peeked out at me. "How do you know about my legs?" she demanded.

Avoiding the daughter card, which I had already ascertained was going to get me nowhere, I stretched the limits of my visual talents. "I could see your legs from the road, Mrs. Colt. They look painful. I would just like to see if you need some help with those sores."

The eye in the doorway studied me up and down. I held my gaze directly on her face. This wasn't my battle, and I wanted her to know it. "Maybe we could get you some salve. I need to look to make sure you don't need antibiotics."

The inquiring eye blinked at me through the cracked door. "What about her? I want her off my porch!"

I looked over at my companion and arched an eyebrow. Her feet shuffled in obvious discontent with the situation. She was used to being in charge, and here I was relegating charge to this diminutive elderly woman whom she considered a nut case. Yet there would be no way she could justify the refusal to let a medical professional examine this woman's legs since that was what the concern from the reporting party addressed. The silence and her battle with the inner workings of her mind were cut short by the eye in the door. "I said that you need to get off my porch so I can talk to this here nurse." Defeat was obvious, and shooting me a glance that said she was not happy with my solution, she reluctantly headed out to the wrought-iron garden bench where the officer had found shade during our exchange.

After watching the departure of our third, I turned back to find Mrs. Colt on my side of the door.

"You really a nurse?" she asked.

"Yes, ma'am, I am." I pulled my county badge free of the clip that held it to my lapel and handed it to her. She wore a cloud of odor around her that spoke of far too few baths and plenty of interaction with the cats. Holding it out away from her face and squinting, she studied it slowly. Finding it to her satisfaction, she returned it to me.

"They're flea bites." Her directness surprised me. "I have a lot of cats, and this time of year, they get fleas. Why are you being nice to me?" she queried.

I smiled. "Why wouldn't I be? I don't know you, and you don't know me. What is there to like or dislike?" I asked.

The wrinkled face turned up to me, and the distrustful eyes took on an amused sparkle. "I like you," she said. "O.K., you can look at my legs." She pulled her well-worn housedress up above her knees. Squatting down, I examined her legs. It appeared she was horribly correct in her evaluation of the sores. They did indeed appear to be flea bites, although the layer of dirt that covered her lower legs hid the flesh that the fleas had somehow feasted on. And they were infected. She needed more than a salve; she did indeed need antibiotics and a good bath!

"Mrs. Colt, these are flea bites, but some of them are infected. This kind of infection can be dangerous. Do you have a doctor?"

"Haven't been in years. Don't trust them."

"Well, Mrs. Colt, I think you need to at least follow up at a clinic. These types of infections can make you really sick. Then who would take care of the cats?" Not really sure where that last question came from, I was nonetheless very happy I had asked it as suddenly Mrs. Colt reached out to me.

"You're not like them." She smiled at me for the first time.

"Mrs. Colt, I'm just here to make sure you're O.K.," I said.

"My name's Emma," she replied. "Been here in this same house my whole life. It's just me and my cats since Fred died. My daughter wants to make me sell and go live in one of those places for old people. Get rid of my cats and sell my house." Her face was somewhere between anger and disbelief that anyone would try to make her do that.

"Well, Emma," I said, once again avoiding the daughter trap, "I think this is a wonderful house. While I was sitting out there in my car waiting for the others, I was imagining how wonderful it must be inside. These old places were made with such love. We just don't let that artistic side of us show in our homes anymore." I looked up at the house and spoke the truth. In spite of that awful odor and the peeling paint, it was a wonderful house.

Emma stepped back and studied me up and down. "You're not going to force me out of my house? It's pretty messy," she said.

"Emma, they can't throw you out of your own house because it is messy," I assured her.

"I suppose you want to see inside?" She asked, looking at me sideways.

"Well, Emma, I'm going to tell you a hard truth now." I looked her straight in the eyes. "One of the reasons all these agencies keep bothering you is because you don't let anyone in your house. You're making it into a mystery, and people always want to solve mysteries."

Emma studied me long and hard. She didn't break eye contact, and neither did I. "I can keep my house no matter how bad it is?" she asked.

"Emma, they may try to make you clean up a little bit if it's really messy, but they can't take your house. You don't seem confused to me." I was getting a little concerned. "Why are you so worried about it? I've seen dirty houses before."

Emma looked down the drive to the shade where the sheriff's officer and the social worker waited. "You make sure they stay put, and I'll show you my house," she said.

Walking down the drive to the two, I told them she had agreed to show me the house if they stayed put. They both looked at me in amazement. "How did you manage that?" I assured them that all I had done was tell her the truth about my purpose for being here.

Emma was waiting on the porch with the door open. The smell of cat urine was overwhelming as the air carried the smell out the door. "I warned you it's messy." Emma looked like she was about to bolt, so I took a deep breath and promised myself that no matter how messy it was, I wouldn't show it. She held the door as I walked in and closed it firmly behind me.

The entryway was dark, and I realized that the fogginess of the windows was not dust but newspapers she had taped over the windows. Slowly my eyes adjusted to the darkness, and slowly the horror of the situation in which Emma lived dawned on me. Gray shadows of cats wound in and out of the furniture, and what looked to be lumps of laundry on the furniture came into focus. The couch took focus first: a wonderful old Victorian sofa with carved wooden legs and arms, and ripped cushions filled with piles of cat feces. The floor was covered with dried piles of excrement, leaving only narrow pathways through the house.

Emma watched my face closely, and I hoped the dim light hid my revulsion. I had earned her trust when no other human had in ten years. I couldn't let her down now. "Wow, Emma, you weren't kidding." I strained against the impulse to cover my mouth as I spoke. "It is pretty messy, but look at that woodwork," I said, looking up at the intricate, cobweb-covered molding and trying to keep myself from gagging.

"Oh," Emma said, filled with delight at her long-awaited houseguest, "wait until I show you the rest!" With that, Emma headed down the feces-framed path to another room, from which flowed a trail of light highlighting the incredible piles of cat leavings. I followed her with trepidation in my heart and found myself in a huge farm kitchen. Indeed, it was quite impressive, with huge cabinets and antique appliances lining the walls—except that every surface was covered in piles of cat excrement. I stared in horror but managed to croak out a positive comment on the antique appliances, asking if they were original.

All health care providers have a place deep inside where they send emotion when it becomes overwhelming. It's a safe place to send their own humanity while they comfort those presenting with whatever horror has triggered the need to escape to that safe place. Traumatic deaths, child abuse, or injuries that would cause a sane person to vomit send the providers' emotional expressions to this safe place. The sane providers—the ones who survive the business—pull all that emotion out after the fact and deal with it away from the patient. That was the place where I sent my response—the part of me that wanted to cover my face and run, to cry, and to puke at the disgusting display before me.

"Aren't they wonderful?" said Emma. "They all work so great that I never replaced any of them. Most of them belonged to my mom." She said with pride, pointing to a wonderful old Wedgewood with a raised light bar that sat in the corner. Only one of the burners, however, would have been serviceable as the rest of the stove was also covered in piles of dried feces. My eyes traveled from there to the entrance of the walk-in pantry, which was no longer walk-in due to the presence of three overflowing litter boxes and piles of feces covering the floor in front of it. I had to force my mind to stay in my safe place and swallowed the gorge that arose at the site of two dead kittens lying on the pile of feces. Emma noticed my focus and started to explain. "Sad," she said. "When the brother and sister kitties have babies, they don't all come out all right."

To say that I was speechless would be the ultimate understatement. I watched in abject horror as a young kitten about the age of the two on the pile wound its way across the kitchen. It had no eyes. The skin over its face was solid fur, and my mind decided that I had stumbled into a stage setting for a Stephen King novel. Somewhere in my safe place I screamed, but on the outside, I smiled at Emma and told her that yes, indeed, that was a very sad fact of nature.

Emma, ever more excited that at last she had human company she could visit with, offered me a cup of coffee. My eyes took in the countertop near the sink where the piles of excrement had been pushed to the back of the cabinets in order to allow for a work surface. That was when the true strength of my denial became apparent as I thanked her profusely and told her that I had just finished two cups and that was my daily limit.

Emma smiled at me. "I have tea too if you change your mind," she said. "I'm almost out but I'm goin' to the store. That is where I was headed when you got here. I take my little wagon up there so I can carry home the cat-food bags. I don't eat much myself."

Emma continued in the spirit of female bonding that she somehow believed we had reached. "Oh, you just have to see my album collection!" she said as she grabbed my arm and led me back through the feces-filled living room and up the stairs to the second floor. I was amazed that even the stairs were covered with filth, except for the narrow footpath that led up to her bedroom and the record album collection she had hoarded for years. Original Doors, Beatles (the dead-baby album cover registered hard), Elvis—priceless in a world that could ignore the hell that surrounded them, the album covers were stapled to the walls and ceilings, which gave my mind a place to escape from the sight of the carved four-poster Victorian bed that was half-covered with filth and hair. The side that Emma slept on was apparent, and I wondered if she swept it all off or just flipped the covers to the other side to clear her sleeping place.

"Emma," my rational side tried, "they might want you to clean this up a bit. I don't think it's very healthy. Do you have a bathroom?"

"Oh, of course," she laughed. "But the bathtub is kind of dirty, and the shower doesn't work." She led me around the corner to see a claw-foot tub that too was half filled with excrement. The pedestal sink was the only area of the bathroom that had somehow survived the onslaught of cat defecation.

"Emma, we need to let that other woman in here. I don't think they will believe me if I tell them about all of this." I knew I spoke the truth. No one was going to believe this. "And Emma, I need to take a few pictures with my phone to show my boss why it took so long to look at your legs."

Emma had accepted my presence, and somehow we had bonded. Years of living with the horror that filled her house had somehow created a strange acceptance and protectiveness in her. "Of course you can take your pictures," she said. "I know the cat shit is everywhere, but that's how me and my cats live. That other gal ain't going to be able to see past the shit."

She was right about that. When I went to the door and called in the social worker, she began to gag at her first sight of Emma's house. Her exit was fast and unexcused. Emma and I wandered through her house again, and I took the pictures I would need for my report. The paranoia at having her secret known had gone and was now replaced by a perverse pride in her strange form of mental illness. I did ask, but she had no idea how many cats she housed and fed. How many cats had it taken to produce what she'd hoarded over the course of ten years? I had no idea.

When we finished the tour for a second time, Emma excused herself, and locking the door behind her, took her little red wagon and began the walk to the store for more cat food. She invited me back for coffee whenever I wanted before she left. I never went.

There is a law on the books in most states called self-determination. Emma knew the condition of her house and chose to live that way. She was injuring no one but herself, and she fully understood the danger that she had created. I told her the truth when I told her that the authorities could not remove her from her home. It turned out that legally they could not even make her clean it out, although I don't believe that anything less than burning that house to the ground would have solved Emma's cleaning problem. They did, however, call in the state livestock bureau. It seems that while sitting on the little bench out front as Emma gave me the grand tour, the sheriff's officer and the representative for APS looked a little more closely at the kittens that were playing in the weeds. Genetic mutations caused by generations of inbreeding had affected more than the little blind, half-dead kitten I had seen in the kitchen. While we were touring her house, the authorities found that, under the cruelty to livestock laws, they could call the Department of Agriculture to remove the badly deformed and sick cats and kittens that shared Emma's existence.

I never went back to check on Emma. Once the authorities removed her beloved cats, she again locked down and wouldn't let anyone near her, including her family. After spreading newspapers over the seats in my county car, I drove to my house in the country and went to my burn barrel. My jacket, scrubs, and even my shoes went into that barrel and were burned. I walked naked into my house and stood in a steaming hot shower until the water ran cold twice. I took the county car back to the office, got in my own car, and went home to a double shot of brandy and another shower. The smell of that house seemed to follow me for days although I don't know how much of that was only in my mind. The photos were turned over to my boss at the health department and added to the archives of weird events.

IT CAN'T HAPPEN TO ME

We had been riding hard in the sun for two hours. My partner, Bob, led on his custom burgundy Road Star with our little dog, Lady, riding behind him in her homemade safety basket. I was riding behind, enjoying the feeling of kicking back and riding drag on my purple Road Star. Deep purple with smooth leather bags and a few female touches of decoration, it was a good bike. Riding was relaxation for me; it gave me a sense of freedom and control.

The sun was blazing hot as we rode the freeway toward home. It had been a long ride. The Reno rally, Street Vibrations, had ended that morning, and the road was filled with bikers headed home. There had been an unusually high number of accidents on the way, dragging the normal three-hour ride out to five, but we were almost home. I was looking forward to a private soak in the tub to erase the road grime.

The gentle vibration of the bike always relaxed me, but this day was dragging on, and the heat was making the ride uncomfortable. Traffic was starting to thin out after we passed Sacramento, which was a relief. Stop-and-go traffic on a motorcycle in the heat was not fun, and I refused to ride the line in traffic this thick. You never knew when someone would decide to change lanes or swerve over without warning.

Adrenaline drowned the fatigue as a small car pulled around us on the right and cut Bob off by inches. I braked and pulled back. Bob yelled—a guy thing, I guess. The person in the car was driving crazy.

Whatever trauma was happening in the bad driver's life exploded because of Bob's yell. The little car jerked to the right, slowing as the driver began a display of the more basic of human emotions.

Slowing more, I pulled to the far side of my lane. More than alarmed by the show of primal force at such a simple stimulus, I gripped my bike firmly and watched as idiocy unfolded in front of me.

I do not remember the full extent of the ride, but I do remember the fear when I realized that the guy in the car was not only chasing us but also swerving in toward us and yelling threats. I panicked when I realized that Bob was responding to the guy's threats. Thinking I had to get to the side of the road and being overwhelmed by guilt that to protect myself, I had to abandon my partner and my dog to road rage, I flicked my right turn signal with my thumb. Checking my mirror, I started to pull to the side. Suddenly abandonment was no longer an issue as the car sped up around on my right and cut in front of me, missing my front wheel by inches.

Time slowed and became surreal as I swerved my bike away from the rear of the vehicle and tried to slow. I watched as the car swung into my lane and butted into Bob's bike in slow motion. The rear wheel caught Bob's boot tip and flipped his leg around in a hideous joke of bone and sinew. He flew off the side of the road, and I knew he was dead. Brake lights—huge round-cornered brake lights flashed directly in front of me. I knew I was down before I hit the brakes. With a semitrailer to the right of me, there was nowhere to go. I remember sliding—sliding on my stomach and thinking I should pull my tank top down as my stomach was being scraped by the road. I remember thinking that I would hurt my hands if I did that and then looking up, seeing sky, and realizing I wasn't moving anymore.

I heard screaming, loud screams of pain. Somewhere my brain registered Bob, and I knew he wasn't dead but hurt. I remember thinking I wasn't dead. I had to get the helmet off my head. Then it was off, but I do not remember where it went. I was walking, and people were telling me to sit down. But I had to help. I was the rescuer, not the patient. Blank spots...I knew somewhere in reality that I had hit my head and tried to assess myself, but I could find no reason in what just happened. Unable to grasp the logic, I needed to pull my mind from the place where it was trapped. I found Bob lying in the grass screaming, his legs twisted in an abstract depiction of the human form. There were people with him, people I did not know. I looked for the dog. "She ran over there." *There* was so far away. My vision tunneled and narrowed when I tried to focus. Miles and miles to *there*. I couldn't walk that far; I had to sit. Bob was still screaming. "Bob, please, shut up. I can't think." They twisted his leg back around to where it should be, and he is yelling louder...

I was in an ambulance then, and I knew these people. They were relatively new to the field. The medic was being so polite, and I didn't want to hurt his feelings. "No C-spine for me, thanks. But O.K., you can start an IV." I couldn't remember much of the ride.

The doors to the back opened, and my son was standing there. They'd called him. He worked for the ambulance company because he was raised around this. I told him I couldn't find the dog, and he said he would look for her. "Don't cry, my son. I'm O.K."

It didn't hurt. They kept asking me if I wanted pain medicine, but it didn't hurt. "Yes, I see the blood. You're right, this should hurt, but it doesn't." Then my son told me that the dog was dead. She'd been fine after the accident but ran from the firefighters. When she tried to get back to me, a car hit her. The medics had watched it happen. I asked him to get her so we could bury her. "Where's Bob?" I can still hear him screaming in pain.

"O.K., give me some morphine. No, I don't hurt, but I'm starting to feel..."

THE OTHER SIDE OF THE GURNEY

For so many years, I worked as a paramedic and a nurse, yet I had never been on the gurney as a patient, never really experienced the other side of the gurney. I taught EMTs to be EMTs, paramedics to be paramedics, and nurses to be nurses. All that time treating, teaching, and saying I knew, yet I didn't really know what it felt like to be on the other side. It is a very different perspective.

I think that it makes me a better nurse that I have been there. Now when I hold the hands of my patients and tell them I know how they feel, I truly do know the shock and the agony of what they are going through. I know how it feels to have tragedy sneak up on you and not be able to find any reason for what happened to help buffer the pain. I know what it feels like to have strangers look at you with pity in their eyes and not understand why. I have felt the helpless feeling of not being able to focus while the adrenaline poured through my veins.

My son quit the ambulance business shortly after this happened. I've never asked him if it had to do with looking in those back doors and seeing his mom. The relationship with the man I was riding with ended a few years after this. He blamed himself for not backing down, and truth be told, so did I. It didn't take a rocket scientist to know that you were going to be on the losing end of a car-versus-motorcycle challenge if you were the one on the motorcycle. It took him two years to be able to walk again, and I don't think his soul ever did heal.

I started riding again after a few years—a Harley Softail this time. I find it to be very relaxing. However, I choose my riding partners with more care, and I am the first to back off if someone on the road is being stupid.

The EMT on the ambulance that took me in was in paramedic school at the time. From what I hear, she turned out to be very good at what she does. I know that the first few times she saw me when I got back to work, we both cried. At the time, I couldn't tell you why in words, but now I think it has to do with realizing the humanity of everyone we touch. Maybe, just maybe, that is one of the reasons she is so good at what she does now.

I certainly would never recommend that caregivers experience firsthand being on the other side of the gurney as a standard of training. I had a very difficult time working emergency for two years after the accident. If I heard on the hospital's EMS radio that a motorcycle accident was coming to our facility, I had to be at the ambulance-bay doors. I had to know who it was, to see their faces. I had to know it wasn't a friend.

For years I had a hard time dealing with brake lights. For a long time, I would dream about them and wake up in a cold sweat. Driving in traffic became a major ordeal, and even though it took years, I am sure that CHP would approve of my safe following distances even to this day.

The man who attacked us was initially charged with attempted manslaughter, but after being held for several months, he was released on a technicality. I heard he is now driving a commercial big rig for a living. Scary thought.

I was able to say thank-you to the people who treated and transported me. They were my heroes that day. I know, even though I don't remember the events fully, that I was probably not an easy patient to deal with. I give them credit for even getting me into an ambulance. From what I learned later, I not only adamantly refused to be in C-spine but also directed the paramedic through the process of cutting off one of my rings, as my hands were terribly disfigured with road rash and a very badly dislocated index finger.

I know that I should have probably died that day. I was driving seventy miles per hour on the freeway on a motorcycle and was attacked by an irate driver who later admitted to the police that he had been fighting with his girlfriend. I believe that God was watching out for me and that somewhere in the greater scheme of things, I still have a purpose here.

Professionally, I now know in my heart what I had learned in my head. I have looked up off that gurney and felt the loss of control and the fear that accompanies it. I have been on the other side of the gurney.

FINALE

W hen I was younger, I believed that the greatest gift one can receive is faith. I prayed for it, believed in the concept, studied the notion, explored the reality, and questioned the validity of the belief in faith as a form of power. I believed my greatest shortfall was a lack of all-encompassing faith in love, in my fellow human beings, in the existence of God, and in the sanctity of life.

Older now, I still believe the truths I found through my search for faith. Faith is not a gift but an understanding. Love is truly amazing when it is shared with someone who returns its treasures. Understanding my fellow human beings makes me more cautious of them but also more accepting. I know there is a God, but I also know that I cannot know his definition of completeness until I understand his creations. And life is indeed sacred; even in its ugliest forms, it serves a purpose.

I know there is love. I have explored the many forms of it. I have felt the intensity of love that allowed me to drown in it and the warmth of love while holding a sleeping child. I have confused it with lust and married it with denial. I have envied the conception and completeness that others have found in it. I have felt the pain of its loss through change, growth, and death. And I have found its completeness in the

st of forms at an age when I know to appreciate it fully. Every
ond of it.

Faith in the sanctity of life does not waver but is buffeted about by
awareness that what sanctifies life is not the same for all. Knowledge
confirms faith, but the growth that supports that knowledge is tur-
bulent, and the process of faith is translucent with the doubts and
questions that are part of the process of that growth. It can become a
frustrating circle if belief in goodness is lacking.

I have had a very interesting life and used to say that I would never
be the old one in the back of an ambulance or on a hospital gurney
bemoaning the wish-I-would-have, wish-I-could-have list. Now I know
that is not true. I will always have things I have not yet done because
the wish list is ever evolving. Life is simply too short, no matter the
span—another proof of the sanctity of life.

I hope you enjoyed this collection of stories. The sad, the happy,
and the silly, they are all true. When I first wrote them, I was concerned with the political correctness of some of them—the references
to the challenges of male and female roles, and the differences between cultures and races. But to deform these stories to make them
politically correct would also remove some of the spice of life. These
are stories that make known the comedies and tragedies of the life
journey of strangers.

Belief in the sanctity of life is the foundation of enjoyment of our
uniqueness and the celebration of lessons learned though the lives of
others. The interspaced reflections of the lessons that I learned serve
as an expression of gratitude to those from whom I have learned
these lessons. I hope you read the stories the way they were written:
as events that unfolded in the lives of others, and lessons learned by
a fellow traveler through intersecting planes of time that are this life.

47150312R00098

Made in the USA
San Bernardino, CA
24 March 2017